ALTRUISTIC DIET (OR WHY ADAM & EVE
STARTED IN THE GARDEN OF EDEN)

ALTRUISTIC DIET (OR WHY ADAM & EVE STARTED IN THE GARDEN OF EDEN)

Michael Perrone Jr.

ISBN-13: 9781977738738
ISBN-10: 1977738737

DEDICATION

First off, I would like to dedicate this book to my Mom & Pops, for their Love, Patience, Affection, Attention and Sacrifices; without which I would not be authoring, this my second (2) book; after-"Cooking for Mom & Pops"...

Also, I would like to dedicate this book to my Dogs; Nicole, Crystal, Chelsea, Luiza & Cookie, whose Dear & Sweet Souls, along with their particular situations compelled me to dig deeper for True Solutions...

Next, I would like to dedicate this work to Mr. Pat Piciano; our insurance professional, whose well timed knock on our door, fifty (50) years ago, was the beginning of half a century of propituous financial advice that was able to provide for my posterior ability to sit here and author this work and concern myself with one-day-at-a-time...

Also, I would like to acknowlege my teachers at Holy Rosary Academy in Union City, NJ; with special Thanks to my fifth grade teacher-Sister Mary Louise- whose quite gentleness has always been an inspiration to me, to this day...

And to my teachers at Saint Joseph's of the Palisades, West New York, NJ;

With Special Thanks to my sophomore biology teacher- Mrs. Diane Krone (nei:Abromoski) who afforded me an extra credit report -"The Double Helix"-by Crick & Watson; beginning my interest in human physiology, which you will noticed in this work and allowed me to pass her class...

And to Father Tom Kenna; the class of '77's Spiritual Advisor, who asked me to attend an Arch-Diocease of Newark"s- Search for Christuan Maturity weekend; where I was later asked to be a Team member and given the -"Good News" talk, because at the interview I akinned the Bible to a novel, a study in history and a book of recipes for life (mainly because I enjoy foods; cooking, but more so eating)...

And to Rafe' Ledesma, whose gift of -"The Little Prince", on my Search weekend and his humanity has been a sextant through out this lifetime...

And also, our principal- Mr. Frank Gargiulo; whose patience with me allowed me to grow into the person I Am (God-Help Us)...

And, Professer "Uncle" Joe Rosen, for being a pal & for introducing me to the Thesis for my nexr book

The various (PBS) Local Public Broadcast Stations; whose many variuos programs of interest have peppered my inspiration and knowledge of the diverse disciplines, which I share with yous, here, within; for which I am donating ten (10%) percent of my proceeds to, with the assurdness that they will continue to inspire posterity.

To Laura, for the gentle smile in her eyes and the melody in her voice...Thank You !!!

And last, but not least, The Eternal Soul, Energy which is the Universe, existence itself; the - "I AM"...

TABLE OF CONTENTS

Have you ever been on a Scavenger Hunt ???

In the 1990's, i was the owner/operator of Bambino's Liquor and Pub, and one of the most fun we had is when I sponsored a local scavenger hunt for my clientele. The Energy & Enthusiasm just filled the place and the people participating.

I have decided to write this work in Re-Verse, mainly because this is a teaching tool, it gets one to go over points in their mind; making this an Active Reading...Most all authors start by teasing their readers with the title, then spend way to many pages (probably, to please their publishers), before they get to the purpose of their writtings.

I am going to do this differently. I am going to start by telling yous, What's - What and spend the rest of the book filling in the Wheres, Whens, Whys, and How...I am also going to use the teaching tool of Re-Iteration, that is repeating a point in different parts of this work, mainly because it fits and also for Re-In-Force-Ment of Learning...

Well...We are about to embark on a Bibical Scavenger Hunt, through various bibles to see if they depict an optimum diet for humanity; while scouring through modern nutritional information, substainiating facts and truths.

Before our very eyes: we will become witness to how the absolut word of God changes with the version of the Bible and acknowledge how man has skewed it for his own purpose. In our day and age, we see the actual proof of this when "Monied Ministers" rewrite the Bible for their own benefit; so as to give more punch to their sermon, lending them authority...so to say.

We will come to an understanding that Divine Inspiration being a spark that glows within us, A spark of Energy that makes up our aura, the aura of our atmosphere (or the very words we read), its vibrations, seen in rainbows, that Benjamin Franklin, understood to exist and grounds us to the very Earth we walk, with its electro-magnetism, a slow vibration of its own, which is damped or magnified by our diets...What we do with it, is our doing. Not so much that - " and God said, let us make man in our own image, after our likeness" (Genisis 1:26); but that we (mankind) have created a God in our own image and likeness !!!

Together we will exculpate the Truth: in the Gospel of John 8:32, Jesus admonishes us -"to seek the truth"; like a diamond in the rough, the Truth, doesn't just present itself; it is an active process. For lies to work, they need a grain of truth.

In this process, we will become - Bibical Palenthologists, bringing us to a better understanding of what is in the bible and why, by combing through the history of the written word. We will read the bible for what it says and what it doesn't say...

All this work to figure out - what Manna from Heaven is??? Yes; that is the road I have been lead on, by the guidance of the Holy Spirit (my mentor), when the question was planted in my thoughts: Is there an optimum diet in the bible, for humanity???

What I did not know was that the foundations for all this was laid just over 40 yrs. ago, in High School when Miss

Abromoski, my sophomore biology teacher, gave me an extra credit report, on the "Double Helix" by Watson & Crick, that allowed me to pass her class. And, by Father Tom Kenna who extended to me an invitation to attend the Archdioceases of Newark, Search for Christian Maturity weekend; where I was eventually asked to give a team talk on the"Good News",(probably because at the interview I akinned the Bible to a cookbook of recipes for individual's lives)...

These have been macerating in my - Little Grey Cells - for 40 years, without my knowing it. The same time frame that a young Galileo Galilei (just think it they had books with popular baby names, way back then) while at church, noticed a swinging chandelier (back then they actually had to light the candels) forty years later, began working on the pendulum mechanism for clocks (giving rise to the stress in our lives over the past five centuries)...

Well...here we are...we are about to answer the questions- "is there an optimum diet for humanity in the Bible and What is Manna from heaven"?

Come on; Let's get this Scavenger Hunt going!!!

CHAPTER 1

IN A NUTSHELL

ANY DIET IS a pattern of eating; so it is obligatory to issue a warning : So Here It Is - WARNING yous should always consult with a proper physician (or doctor for the layman); preferably a Natruopathic doctor who can perform a proper Bio-Nutritional Analysis (BNA)- as I also recomended in my first book (in my triology) -"Cooking for Mom & Pops"- that will point out your own personal strengths and weaknesses, that you can then properly tailor your nutritional intake for. Makes sense; Ahey!!!

Now our second WARNING is that a holistic or naturopatic doctor, is just as human as the rest of them. I learned this the hard way with the holistic vet I used for my two dogs; Chelsea & Luiza. He was fine when it came to nutritional advice; but when doing procedures, would gloss over the obvious, to the determent of my sweat-hearts, costing them their lives; anguish and heart-ache for us all...So, do your home-work and do not rely totally on some one else; use your BNA as a guide for your pesonal health. Keep your instincts sharp and play it by ear !!!

So-MANY people put the cart before the horse; taking so many suplements and skewing their diets, for a presumed purpose, that 98% fail yearly. Mega-dossing supplements (also, Vegetable oil & shortening) can lead to - plasticosis, a built up of plastic in your system, because you can not digest, nor eliminate the plastic coating on the capsules. It's just to much...

I take fish oil supplements because I am not a fish eater, some tuna from a can, once per month is tops for me. Well, I decide to switch fish oil supplements from a reputable company to the company I order my supplements from. I begin getting an oily build up in my ear; I'm thinking some thing is going on. My fish oil supplements run out so I wait a week or two to order, because I did not have a need for anything else. Well, don't you know, the oily build up in my ear disappears; I was swabbing my ears twice a day. Just goes to show that sometimes, by mistake, the right thing happens...

Okay, now for the hypothisis - Is there an optimum diet for humanity in the Bible ? The answer is : YES !!! It is - Vegetables and Legumes, with some Meat and Fruits (Fresh & Dried) with Nuts...By some meats I mean a few slices, because a pound of meat averages 2,000 calories. Okay, there are many a people who have nut allergies, so you may wish to swap-out the nuts for seeds; you should sprout them, because eating seeds with the shells still on them, makes about as much sense as eating the nuts with the shells still on then (DO NOT TRY THIS !!!)...Think of corn kernals, on the cob, as you bite into them they burst through their protective coating and the next day, you will usually see many floating in the bowl...

Next - What is Manna from Heaven ? ?? Which is the proper filler for humanity, so as not to be continually hungry...The answer is - LENTILS; specifically Yellow Lentils, which have a reddish interior and we will come to see, that the Bible tells us so (in many more words than I would of like to have read)...

LENTILS: for which Esau (Jacob's twin brother) gave up his birthright for a pottage of; that the Hebrews were sustained on their meandering by; that combined with a vegetarian diet can increase one's countainence by, as Daniel and his friends; that may just be the gateway or portal to the Seventh (7) Sense; and may have been the special concotion the Comte de Saint Germain subsisted on that increased his longevity or centuries ???

I was extatic once I came to the realization that LENTILS were Manna from Heaven. In all their forms, LENTILS are a nutrionally versatile powerhouse. Containing a good amount of dietary fiber, soluble and insoluble, and lean protein, alkalizing the body's ph, along with Iron and folate makes it a real winner in a healthful healing diet for approximately 13,000 years, especially in the Near East where it is indiginous to and we are sticking our noses into...

I was reading a piece about the Seventh Sense and inadvertantly (and without knowing it) there is mention in the very first line of how when young and hard pressed the family often ate -LENTILS - for supper and I'll bet much vegetables, also...

THIS IS A SIMPLE DIET, BUT NOT AN EASY ONE !!!

Now, there yous have it; go off now and be Happy!!! Yous don't even have to read the rest of this book; unless yous want to know and understand the Why, What, Where, When and How I have come to this??? In the mean time, I will give yous a basic recipe for making Lentil-bread, which is your daily filler.

- For each person; get a Omer (or Liter, which I will explain later as I develop my thesis) of Lentils, soak in a bowl of water for three (3) to four (4) hours or even up to a day, which begins sprouting and activating DNA and enzymes; over night to a day is even better...

- Next; drain water through collander or shive and shake about (not you, the Lentils) to eliminate more water (you don't want a soggy product); and place in a food processor or mortar and pestal (if you want to work out some fustrations), or even a fork to smouch with, and add approximately three (3) tablespoons of baking powder.

Yes, the Israelites did have access to baking powder; it is yeast they are not suppose to use, because when activated by water, yeast becomes a living organism and not acceptable for sacrifices. (You want it to hold together like a meatloaf-if it is soggy put it in a cheese cloth and squeeze or if dry add a little moisture)...

It is interesting to me how trial and error was used through out many a millenium. Bibical or ancient bakers had access to Baking Powder; made of Baking Soda, obtained from ashes of plants, and Cream of Tartar, which was a crude substance adhearing to the sides of wine casks. What an elongated process...How long do yous think it took someone to figure this out??? It's not as if they had a cook book to reference...Much easier to go to the local market !!!

Once you get use to the proper texture, which you will recognize after a few times, you can bake in an oven 350 to 375 degrees; dependent on your oven and container you use to bake...We have many diverse containers, or baking pans, to choose from. I like using a silicon bundt pan ; there are others - loaf pans, muffin pans, corn cake pans...and bake for 20 to 45 minutes, which depends on the temperature and the style of baking pan you use...You will have to experiment a few times and once you get it correct, write it down-you'll know it's correct, when you can draw out a tooth-pick dry (the time-tested bakers' method)...And here you have it...

If you wish your lentil bread - savory, add some dried herbs and when finished baking, you can drizzle some olive oil over it. If you add olive oil to the mixture (pre-baking), it may be to muschy and may not bake well. If you wish a sweet product, you may add honey to the mixture, but you'll have to eye-ball it, because this too may break down your product. I perfer to to drizzle and/or smear some honey over the product.

You may also cold-bake...What is this ??? Actually quite simple...Ya see when one boils the Lentils, one reduces the protien content; hence baking, as I have described, is prefer-rable... Now, (get ready for -Nutrition 101) in legumes there is a Phytatic shell (like on our kernal of corn) - a very thin covering that keeps all the DNA (look at us being fancy) or the essence of the seed together. Of course, the bigger the seed the bigger the shell, like a walnut...It is water or mois-ture that begins the germinating process and if left to long in hot climate, ferments. This is why seeds found in tombs, in desert regions, dating back 30,000 years, were still intack; once planted, yielded a plant...Just think, what it is like to wait 30,000 years to yawn and stretch up to the sun...Also why sque-riels bury their nuts, to allow them to germinate and break through their shell, making the nuts easier to eat...WOW; look at this knowledge we are imparting !!!

For all you - Die Hard - bread people; whom just can-not give up Bread - I have a compromise solution...Yes, yous can have your Bread and eat-it-too !!! Sprout the grains and make it yourself (WE-OK-KEE)...In the next chapter, where I men-tion Manna, that it lay with the morning dew - moisture, which takes time., but was a more common practice. With all the added peoples, some Hebrew probably got the bright idea to mash & bash the grain into a flour and then bake or boil, with honey or olive oil as additions (probably the first bagels)...

As a tangent, since we are speaking of sprouting; What about rice ??? Rice is a seed, if yous wash your rice, which means soak it in water over night to a full day, you will extract the starch (that white milky stuff, that gets into our systems and causes Havoc, which we will speak of in a later chapter) and yous may serve it up as you like as a filler. Washing the rice is the reason that Orientals stay slim & trim and we Westerners get bloated. I learned this trick many years ago while picking up a Doctor of Accupuncture for a client of mine, when I opperated a limousine service. The family was having breakfast and eating rice; I happened to noticed a large bowl, on the counter top, of white milky stuff and inquired. I was given the answer, I have just shared with yous...

Well, now you all can become Master-Bakers (be nice) and make your own Sprouted Bread. In sprouting the grain you will be activating its DNA and in doing so, making the product more bio-availible to you. You may wish to get a book on Sprouting or look it up on-line. The basics are this: choose your grain(s), choose a jar large enough to make a loaf of Bread from, place grain in jar, add spring water, secure a lid that is ventilated, let sit for a day or two or three, (don't forget to change the water) dependending on the grain you've selected (hence a book would be more explainitary). Drain through a catch screen, you may rinse, if yous wish.

(Wheter you add more water or yeast or baking powder or herbs, should be in a mixing bowl - honey you may drizzle or dunk into when done)...Follow usual Bread Baking procedures...

Also, you can pan-fry your bread on the stove-top by preparing a large no-stick pan with olive oil, I like a medium flame, let the pan get hot, then pour your mixture in, then cover with a lid. You may wish to splash some water around the edges to develop a moist baking environment. Flip, in ten minutes, then let it cook for another ten minutes or until done. Baking is the same as if you were baking a loaf of Bread normally- temperature & time...

Now back to our show and Cold Baking!!! Have yous ever made Herbal Butter or Fois-Gras ??? This is the same comcept. Soak your Lentils, up to a day (if you like), drain water and place in food processor or use a fork. This is the moment to decide if you want sweet or savory ??? Add Honey for sweet or seasoning, spices, etc., if you want savory - spin to desired texture. Line a pan with plastic wrap, brush with olive oil for savory, with butter or not if you want sweet, place Lentils in pan, fold over the remaining plastic wrap, then place in the refridgerator for a day or until it sets up firm... When ready to eat, take out of fridge (or climb in with knife & fork), but first, open plastic wrap, place a dish over pan, invert, pull pan away, peel away plastic wrap, slice and Mangia (or eat) !!!

Now, the real Queation : Is this diet practical and/or pragmatic ??? Yes and No !

Yes; if you live wiithin walking distance of a Fruit & Vegetable market, with no other food source within a thousnd (1,000) miles, and No; because of all the food temptations in your supermarket, on the road ways, on TV; heck, in our day & age we can even get temptation delivered to us, even Via-App... THIS DIET IS SIMPLE; NOT EASY !!!

So, now yous understand why Jesus had to go into the dessert to fast; he would never had made it forty (40) days in Jerusalem; and he was Jewish; just think it he was from an Italian household, like myself, who sufferd (as I still do) through all the culinary "P"'s : Pasta, Patate, Pane, Pizza, Provolone, Pastries, Panetone - Jesus, would not have a snowball's chance in Hades. My Mom, cooked so wonderfully; that when my relations would come for Christmas Eve & Day celebrations, we never had to wash the dishes, because they would eat those too.

So, why have I chosen to write about this divine diet - an Epiphiny ??? Well, kinda; ya see about seven (7) years ago I experienced a miracle, well at least for me. I lost 36 pounds in six (6) weeks. I decide for a six (6) week period I would be a vegetarian (what's life without a little whimsy), but without Bread (this is wear Vegetarians & Vegans make their mistake)...

Many renowned people in history were vegetarians. One of our most notably was Benjamin Franklin, who, because of reasons of frugality (less expensive - "a penny saved is a penny earned) was a vegetarian in the early part of his life. After leaving (or excaping) his older brother's servitude (indentured servant) as a printing apprentice, Ben Franklin made it to Philadelphia, were walking into town, the first day, he carried a big smile and two (2) loaves of Bread under his arm... (Just think if Ben knew then what I know now!!!)

At the time I was already riding my bicycle for twelve (12) miles per day and not losing an ounce of wieght. Within the first few days of beginning the vegetarian diet, I could sense changes occuring. The most noticable was that my energy level rose; by the end of the six (6) weeks riding my bicycle was not longer a chore, twelve (12) miles was a breeze and I sailed up hills, I had previously labored to climb. I needed less sleep and awoke refreshed.

There is a few reasons for energy increase under this type of diet. First off, you are filling up with good quality nutrition. Star-date: 2017, for the past decade, or so, most all dietary programs have focused on fruits, vegetation, legumes and nuts; wheter in solid or liquid form. We will get into the why's in a later chapter. Good fuel, means good performance.

Number two (2); which is what we're discussing, here. Human beings do not have the Enzymes to digest - Grains (this is where Vegetarians & Vegans make their mistake); which is what we normally put into our mouths to fill our tummies, and usually takes approximately 18 to 24 hrs. to get through our system and emerge out the other end. Also, in a later chapter, we will discuss what happens on this daily journey. The increase in fiber, due to this more natural diet, makes for smooth sailing of approximately 4 to 6 hours; hence allocating less energy for digestion and allowing more for your body's usage.

Thirdly, there is a tremendous amount of energy in fat-storage. As the body begins to release, then burn the stores of fat, the latent energy in reserve gets released; along with the toxins that are stored in fat reserves, Hence it is why an increase of fluids is desirable, to help in the flushing out of the body of all the icky-gunk that the body accumulates over time.

One does have to adjust their fluid intake, because of the fresh fruit uptake, you will be urinating more. A simple rule of tumb is ; puffiness under the eyes - to much fluids; swollen ankles - not enough fluids (as long as there no other medical reason for each). I would suggest dried fruits in the later part of your day, so as to avoid excess urination over-night. Did you know that it was common for ancient man (before central heating), to arise during the evening to stoke the fires so as to maintain a warm domicile and while up, practice writting ones name in the snow.

So, what's the down side ??? Always hungry... So, I began looking for the optimum filler, that was not one of the "P's", I had become depended on over the past fifty (50) years. And so, like so many before me, who when pondering -Life's Great Questions- I turned to the Bible and Divined upon - Manna...

In the mean time, I'm sure yous have heard the phrase - "the best laid plans of mice or men, do often go awry"; which boils down to, no matter what yous do, a monkey wrench will always show up in the works. Yous can have everything planned out and something may be missing.

I hate, walking around the house saying to myself - "I want something; I just don't know what it is"...This is called a Craving (for you lay folk & intellectuals alike) and can be a valuable guide to what your body needs, if yous understand it...

Or some one may pop-up, out-ta nowhere, with something irrestible to you and yous just can't say - NO !!! Or an event gets past you and now you are stuck looking at tables of wonderful FOODS.

Well, let me share some of my CHEATS with you. When I'm wandering, I follow a Star and my Star is Chocolat. I Love Chocolat; but Chocolat does not Love me; I ate a brownie and a lump apeared by my ankle, so a small piece or square with some nuts usually does da trick. You may even splurge on some nuts or raisins or other dried fruit covered in Chocolat.

Yous can even let it sit in your moist mouth and melt down your throat, so as to inebriate your taste buds.

For the unexpected visit or visitor, I'll make a small vegetable salad with some pieces of meat,(we digest best, what we ingest first) and fill up on quality, before walking down the path of temptation; hence, indulging in less of the temptation.

And for the - Soiree' Irrestible - I use a dieter's tea (not to be mis-used, because it may cause pancreatic problems). DON'T over eat; eat sensibly or smartly, subcome to temptation, if you must (the Venetian table does me in) and have a dieter's tea in the evening, which will aid in evacuating your bowels in the morning. This is just a crutch to lean on once-in-awhile; NOT Always... Life is too short to live in a box or deprive one self of all the sins; even Jesus allowed the Apostles to Woop-It-Up some and at the wedding in Cana, he turned the water into wine (it would of been a greater miracle, if he'd turn the Water into Cola...)

Now let 's talk about some recipes to help yous out some, all of which should be accompanied by your special Lentil (Manna) Bread...How's-bout a - Fritz Salad ??? Fairly simple; a nice large bowl filled with your favorite vegetation. The variety of greens & mixed vegetables makes this a cornicopia of variables. Yous can go a whole month without repeating the same combination. Now add a few pieces of your favorite meat or some eggs (for the more orthodox, you should use diverse softened legumes)... If you are weight conscious and looking after them calories, keep in mind that a pound of meat is approximately 2,000 calories. A simple trick I use is I'll purchase a pound of, let's say, roast beef which usually comes to 20 slices; so 5 slices would be 500 calories or 100 calories per slie. See, simple ! Vinegars are excepional in cleansing the arteries & viens of built up - gunk, and there are so many available, that every salad can be a welcomed surptise. V-I-O-L-A; yous have a menu item.

Another simple dish, I enjoy, needs a frying pan, over medium heat, some olive oil & a tab of butter, place a sausage (or some other meat in) to saute'... Cut up a medium sweet potato, and put it in, cover with a lid. Half way through, I'll cut up the sausage or meat, so as to cook evenly with the sweet potato; at the end you can add some spinach or other chiffonaded greens (if you choose kale, you should massage the leaves first and cut the rib out and save for a soup). When done, scoop out into a bowl, leaving as much oil behind. Now crack in 2 or 3 eggs, a splash of water and cover with the lid until cooked; then slide onto your potato and sausage or meat. Cut up everything, then shovel into the mouth; YUM !!! (Don't Forget to start with a nice mixed vegetable salad and use your Lentil Bread to shovel...)

How's-bout a soup ??? I'll purchase rotissere chicken for my dogs and save the juice in a one pound container, when full, I use this as my stock. Place in a pot over medium heat & add 2 containers of water and some tomato sauce (always season at the end). Chop up some shallots (these are higher up the nutrition chart) and add in some frozen mixed vegetables. Then i'll take a shower, by the time I'm finished my concoction is boiling, season, close heat, place lid on and let sit for 5 to 10 minutes. Yous can add some cut up green leafy vegetables for a minestra or add some legumes, from a can, for a minestrone. Sometimes I will whisk in some eggs; making this an egg-drop-vegetable soup and slice up some Manna-Lentil Bread, maybe a smear of jam (makes life a little sweeter) !!!

What about a soup made with your favorite Gords ??? Take your favorite, or mix them up; pumpkin, squashes, zuc-ca-ninni (zucchine), cucumbers, what ever is available or in season. Cut them open, take out the seeds (yous can plant them when the season is right and have your own Squash-Garden), seperate from the skin, cut then into chunks and place in a nice sized pot leaving space, about a quarter of the pot, to the top. Cover your Squash with water or broth of choice, place lid on pot and turn up da heat, until it boils; turn heat to medium, then cook until soft. In the mean time yous can crisp up some bacon or prosciutto or thin slices of deli meat in the oven or in a skillet or pick apart some left over meats or if you're looking for a more vegetarian version, get a can of your favorite beans ready. Now, take an immersion blender to your Squashes and let-er-rip, nice n'smooth or chunky, as you like. Laddle into a bowl, season as you like, place your meat or legume of choice on top, accompany with your Lentil-Bread and don't forget to start with a salad...VIOLA !!!

For something quick, I like a can of French cut beans, water drained, in a pan with olive oil, garlic and red pepper flakes and some shredded meat, like chicken or turkey, add some fresh spring water and while everything is cooking over a medium flame, make a nice salad of your preference. Once the water as evaporated, you can add some nuts or not, letting it sit for a few minutes. You may spoon it over your salad or serve in a seperate bowl...YUM-YUM !!!

Here's my third WARNING- eating healthy can be injurious...What do I mean ??? I was eating a nice salad, with tomatos, mixed vegetables, olives, beans and chomping away, I hear and feel a CRACK in my rear moller. Apparently, the tip of an olive pit was left behind...OUCH !!! Another time, I had just returned and was chomping down some walnuts; loe & behold, one of those rascals slid between my upper & lower front teeth and SNAP; I lost the front upper tooth and I am still missing it to this day, as a reminder...

My Chelsea had developed a growth on her rear leg from the fatty end of a piece of cooked salmon, so I began giving her some goat's milk, which is closets to human milk, in enzymes, with her meal. Being that goat's milk does not have along shelf life, I was making pudding for myself. Even though the goat's milk seemed to be reducing the growth, by the end of a month we were both experiencing disorientation.

A few years before, I had come upon a raw diet for dogs; seemed reasonable to feed them species appropriate foods. Well, Chelsea had no problems with it; but my Luiza cracked a tooth and developed a lump, a fatty cyst, on her head, probably couldn't digest a hunk-a-fat... A raw diet depends on a fresh kill, so if you do not have a butcher, near by, that kills live animals, then the product one purchases in the stores has already been frozen and refrigerated, which means the vitality has left and the fat congealed...So, take your time and be careful and conscientious of what you are putting in your mouth and that of your Loved-Ones...I advocate, cooked food for dogs the bones are softer and the fat is soliable, rare to medium rare, no more than 120 degrees, keeps the enzymes intack.

How's about a ni-za sanga-wych (as they say in my family) or sandwich, for us land lovers. But you said no bread !!! And I meant it !!! What I do is, normally I like romaine lettuce. but you can use what ever green leaf you desire. Lay out two or three leafs on top of each other, lay out whatever meat you choose, I like roast beef, with smear of mayo, for me, or you can use a hummus of your choice or even an olive spread. I enjoy some roasted peppers, you can also use tomatos, pickles, etcetera. Build it as you wish, you can fold it, taco style, or top it with two more leafs of your lettuce and make a sandwich.

A variation on this is the bun-less burger, iceberg lettuce works nice with this, maybe a fried egg with the yolk pierced, cheese, if you pleaze...Are you in the mood for - ROLLETINI ??? I like a softer letuce for this, like Boston lettuce. One or two leafs, open them up, put your choice within, roll it up and pick a dipping sauce...I like mustard or tomato sauce for meats; mayo for poultries; maybe some oil & garlic for seafood...Go Nutz...You know, make it Nice !!!

Have yous ever made Hummus ??? It's real simple...I take a can of beans, red kidney, white cannellini, chich peas (the standard), any beans you like, yous can mixed them up some... Drain out the water, place in a food processer (or use a fork to smoosh them), drizzle in some olive oil, add garlic, I like red pepper flakes, some parsley, or other seasoning yous like and give it a wurl...You can use it as a dressing or a spread or a snack...HHmmm; HHmmm !!!

Have you ever had a real Pasta Primavera ??? Which is a misnomer, because Primavera means Spring, in English, and in Spring there are only flowers, seeds and dirt. In truth, this should be called - Pasta del Autunno, or Autumn Pasta, in English, because all the vegetation is flourishing in late Summer and early Autumn.

So, for Pasta del Autunno; make your favorite tomato sauce, as you wish, add a variety of vegetables, soon as it's ready you add in some Spiralized Squash and put on the lid, shut of the fire. In a few minutes - ats sa done!!!

We are so fortunate to live in the 21st Century, one in which there is a gizmo or gadget for anything and everything.

There's Blenders, there's Food Processers, there's Bread makers. there's this, there's that and what-nots...To accompany all this there are a pletora of books & information on how-to do anything.

I suggest yous look into them, to keep things mixed up and interesting. You should make the effort to check out my - Bibliography - at the end of this book; where you can examin the list of sources I went through in formulating my thoughts for the Altruistic Diet... Even though adaptability is the main stay of our evolution; we humans, tend to dig ourselves into a SECURITY-RUT...Yes; You & Me; We Be Victims of HABIT...

DA BIBLE VERSES DA BIBLE

DID YA SEE what I did in the title of this chapter ? Instead of using versus, to show opposition I used verses because I will be pitting bible verses against bible verses from the -in this corner, the Good News (GN); in the opposite corner, the American Catholic (ACB); in that corner, the American Standard (ASB) and in the other corner, the King James Bible (KJV). It's a good thing I do not have anymore bibles, because I've run out of corners.

We will begin to see how the absolut word of God- morphs, (words are the greatest source of misunderstanding) depending who and when it was penned. This morphing got me ta thinking; so I began a journey looking into the history of the old testament, the new testament and even the written word; Very Interesting !

If I were you; I would read a section and then pause to think of what the similarities are and more important what they are not...Especially when yous get to Exodus 16; this is where my little grey cells began to perculate...

OLD TESTAMENT
Genesis 1:29 & 30

(KJV) And God said,"I have given you every herb bearing seed which is upon the face of the all the earth and every tree in the which is the fruit of a tree yielding seed; to you it shall be as meat. And to every beast of the earth and to every fowl of the air and to every thing that creppeth upon the earth, where in their is life, I have given every green herb for meat."

(GN) I have provided all kinds of grains and all kinds of fruit for you to eat; but for all the wild animals and all the birds, I have provided grass and leafy plants to eat...

(ASB) and God said,"behold I have given you every plant yielding seed which is upon the face of the earth and every tree, with seed in its fruit, you shall have then for food. And every beast of the earth and to every bird of the air and to everything that creeps on the earth, everything that has the breath of life, I have given every geren plant for food.

(ACB) God also said,"see I give you every seed bearing plant all over the earth and every tree that has seed bearing fruit on it, to be your food. And all the animals of the land, and all the birds of the air, and all the living creatures that crawl on the ground, I give all the green plants for food.

Comment: We are before the fall from God's Grace here; in the GN, we see grains for humans, where the others give us vegetables, fruits & nuts as meat and the animals get grass & herbs... (probably why Adam had a clear relationship with God)...

Genesis 3:19

(KJV) In the sweat of thy face shall thou eat bread, till thou return to the ground.

(GN) You will have to work hard and and sweat to make the soil produce anything, until you go back to the soil from which you were formed; you were made from soil and you will become soil again.

(ASB) In the sweat of your face you shall eat bread till you return to the ground, for out of it you were taken; you are dust and unto dust you shall return.

(ACB) By the sweat of your face you will get bread to eat, until you return to the ground from which you were taken, For you are dirt and unto dirt you shall return.

Comments: This is after the fall from God's Grace and it looks like BREAD is suppose to be a punishment (apparently God never had a loaf of fresh, warm, just out of the oven Italian Bread)...It is also interesting, to me, being a student of history; that Grains are subsidized in our day & age. Subsidized, back to the times of the Romans, where a young Julius Ceaser, was know to give away Bread to his constituents. Subsidized back to the time of the Hebrews - People came from all over the world to buy grain from Joseph, because the famine was severe everywhere... (Genesis 41:57)...Also, interesting to note here, that nutrition is in the soil; from whence we came and are to return to...

Genesis 9:2 & 3

(KJV) Every moving thing that liveth shall be meat for you, even as the green herbs have I given you all things.

(GN) All the animals, birds and fish will live in fear of you. They are all placed under your power. Now you can eat them, as well as green plants; I give them all to you for food.

(ASB) Every moving thing that lives shall be food for you, and as I gave you the green plants, I give you everything.

(ACB) Every creature that is alive shall be yours to eat; I give them all to you as I did the green plants.

Comment: Here we are, after Noah's flood and it looks like God is expanding the menu,(40 days & nights on a boat is a long time; maybe they jumped the gun and Bar-Be-Qued ???)

Genesis 25:34

(KJV) Then Jacob gave Esau bread and pottage of lentils, and he did eat and drink and rose up and went his way; thus Esau despised his birthright.

(GN) Then Jacob gave him some bread and some soup. He ate, drank, got up and left.

(ASB) Then Jacob gave Esau bread and pottage of lentils; he ate and drank, got up and went his way. Thus Esau despised his birthright.

(ACB) Jacob then gave Esau some bread and lentil stew. Esau ate, drank, got up and went his way. Esau cared little for his birthright.

Comment: We see here the first mention of Lentils, in the bible; apparently important enough to give up one's birth-right (mighty tasty them Lentils is...)

Exodus 2:15,16 & 21

(KJV) But Moses fled from the face of Pharoh and dwelt in the land of Midian. Now the priest of Midian had seven daughters...And Moses was content to dwell with them and he gave Moses his daughter Zipporah.

(GN) When the King heard about what had happened, he tried to have Moses killed, but Moses fled and went to live in the land of Midian...So Moses decided to live there and Jethro gave him his daughter, Zipporah in marriage.

(ASB) When Pharoh heard of it, he sought to kill Mosses. But Moses fled from Pharoh and stayed in the land of Midian and he sat down by a well.

(ACB) Pharoh, too, heard of the affair and sought to put him to death. But Moses fled from him and stayed in the land of Midian.

Comment: If I don't miss my guess - looks like Moses went to live in Midian (this is important because Midian is present day Saudi Arabia, which Moses probably went back to when he had the Hebrews in tow).

Exodus 3:11

(KJV) Now, Moses kept the flock of Jethro, his father-in-law, the priest iof Midian and he led the flock to the backside of the desert and came to the mountain of God, even to Horeb.

(GN) One day, when Moses was taking care of the sheep and goats of his father-in-law, Jethro the priest of Midian, he led the flock across the desert and came to Sinai, the holy mountain.

(ASB) Now Moses, was keeping the flock of his father-in-law, Jethro, the priest of Midian and he led his flock to the west side of the wilderness and came to Horeb, the mountain of God.

(ACB) Meanwhile Moses was leading the flocks of his father-in-law Jethro, the priest of Midian. Leading the flock across the desert, he came to Horeb, the mountain of God.

Comment: Moses is still in Midian (Saudi Arabia) when he takes a walk with the sheep to Mt.Sinai (which we've been told to be in Egypt; apparently - NOT SO...)

Exodus 16:13.14,15,16,22,31,32 & 35

(KJV) And it came to pass at even quails came up and covered the camp and in the morning the dew lay round about the host... And when the dew that lay was gone up, behold upon the face of the wilderness there lay a small round thing as small as the hoar frost on the ground...And when the children of Israel saw it, they said one to the another; it is Manna, for they wist not what it was. And Moses said to them, this is the bread which the Lord hath given you to eat... This is the thing which the Lord hath commanded. Gather of it every man according to his eating, an omer for every man, according to the number of your persons, take ye every man for them which are in the tents...And the house of Israel called the name thereof Manna; and it was like corriander seed, white and the taste of it was like wafers made with honey... Bake that which you will bake today, seethe that which you will seethe...Fill an omer of it to be kept for your generations that they may see the bread wherewith I have fed you in the wilderness...And the people of Israel did eat Manna, forty years, until they came unto the borders of the land of Canaan...

(GN) In the evening a large flock of quail flew in, enough to cover the camp, and in the morning there was dew all around the camp...When the dew evaporated, there was something thin and flaky on the surface of the desert. It was as delicate as frost... When the Israelites saw it they did not know what it was and asked each other;"what is it?" Moses said to them,"this is the food that the Lord has given you to eat,,,The Lord has commanded that each of you is to gather as much of it as he needs, two quarts for each member of the household...Bake today what you want to bake"...The people of Israel called the food Manna. It was like a small white seed and tasted like thin cakes made with honey... Moses said,"the lord has commanded us to save some Manna to be kept for our descendants, so they can see the food He gave us to eat in the desert"...That the Israelites ate Manna for the next forty years, until they reached the land of Canaan...

(ASB) In the evening quail came up and covered the camp, and in the morning dew lay about the camp...And when the dew had gone up, there was on the face of the wilderness a fine, flake like thing, fine as hoar frost on the ground...When the people of Israel saw it they said to one another,"what is it?" For they did not know what it was. And Moses said," It is the bread that the Lord has given you to eat"...This is what the Lord has commanded,"gather it every man of you, as much as you can eat; you shall take an omer a piece, according to the number of persons whom each of you has in his tent...Bake what you will bake and boil what you will boil...And Moses said,"this is what the Lord has commanded,"Let an omer of it be kept throughout your generations, that they may see the bread I fed you in the wilderness"...Now the house of Israel called its name Manna; it was like coriander seed, white and the taste of it was wafers made with honey...

(ACB) In the evening quail came up and covered the camp. In the morning, dew lay all about the camp...And when the dew evaporated, there on the surface of the desert were fine flakes like hoar frost on the ground...On seeing it, the Israelites asked one another,"what is this?" For they did not know what it was. But Moses told them,"this is the bread the Lord has given you to eat...Now, this is what the Lord has commanded. So, gather it that everyone has enough to eat, an omer for each person, as many of you as there are, each man providing for each in his tent...You may either bake or boil the manna as you please"...The Israelites called this food Manna, it was like coriander seed, but white and it tasted like wafers made with honey... Moses said,"This is what the LORD has commanded. Keep an omerful of Manna for your descendants, that they may see what food I gave to eat in the desert...The Israelites ate this Manna for forty years, until they came to settled land, they ate Manna until they reached the borders of Canaan...

Comment; Here we have the first mention of Manna, the componants of which is telling. There is dew, which evaporates (which also means there was water or moisture for sprouting). There is a residue which looks like hoar-frost (probably sprouting ???). There is gathering of an omer. there is boiling (maybe the first bagels) and baking. There is a a comparison to corriander seeds. There is a taste of honey. There is a geogarphical ending of their supply. Very Interesting !!!

Also, dew (water, moisture) is very important, in that it provides a mechanism for sprouting... When I walk my dogs, the dew starts accumulating in the evening and by morning, the dew is so heavy, that my boots soak through, so as my socks get wet. Laying seed out, at night, would begin its sprouting & softening...In the Fall, I notice, that on the grass is finely woven, white silky strands (Hoar-Frost ???), which spiders weave to capture the inspects that are snuggling into the ground before winter starts. This would seem to corroborate my thought that the Hebrews laid their LENTILS out over night with moisture...

Nimbers 11:7,8 & 9

(KJV) And the Manna was as coriander seed and the color therof as the colour of bdellium...And the people went about and gathered it in mills or beat it in a mortar and baked it in pans and made cakes of it and the taste of it was as fresh oil...and when the dew fell upon the camp in the night, the Manna fell upon it..

(GN) Manna was like small seeds, withish-yellow in color...It fell on the camp at night, along with the dew. The next morning the people would go around, gather it, grind it or pound it into flour and then boil it and make it into flat cakes...It taste like bread baked with olive oil...

(ASB) Now the Manna was like coriander seed and its appearance was like bdelluium...The people went about and gathered it in mills or beat it in mortars and boiled it in pots and made cakes of it ; the taste of it was like cake baked with oil...

(ACB) Manna was like coriander seed and had the appearance of bdellium...When they had gone about and gathered it up, the people would grind it between mill stones or pound it in a mortar, then cook it in a pot and make it into loaves, which tasted like cakes made with oil...At night when the dew fell upon the camp, the Manna also fell...

Comment: WHAT-DA-HEY ??? ; maybe yous should read Numbers, again... Here we have the comparison of Manna to coriander seed, with the addition of bdellium, which is a reddish color (rust-like or orangey); also pounding and beating into a flour, making cakes with olive oil.

Levitcus 2:11

(KJV) No meat offering which ye shall bring unto the Lord, shall be made with leaven; for ye shall burn no leaven, nor any honey, in any offering to the Lord made by fire...

(GN) None of the grain offerings which you present to the Lord, may be made with yeast; you must never use yeast or honey in food offering to the Lord...

(ASB) No cereal offering which you bring to the Lord shall be made with leaven; for you shall burn no leaven, nor any honey, as an offering, by fire, to the Lord...

(ACB) Every cereal offering you present to the Lord shall be unleavened for you shall not burn any leaven or honey as an oblation to the Lord...

Comment: Here, the Hebrews are still wandering, yet they have grain offering and yeast (for leavening) and honey available to them, (I guess this is where matza came in handy)...

Joshua 5:11 & 12

(KJV) And the Manna cease on the morrow after they had eaten of the old corn of the land; neither had the children of Israel Manna any more, but they did eat of the fruit of the land of Canaan that year...

(GN) the next day was the first time they ate food grown in Canaan; roasted grain and bread made without yeast. The Manna stopped faling then and the Israelites no longer had any...

(ASB) And the Manna cease on the morrow when they ate of the produce of the land ; and the people of Israel had Manna no more, but ate of the fruit of the land of Canaan that year...

ACB) On the day after the Passover they ate of the produce of the land in the form of unleavened cakes and parched grain. On that day after the Passover on which they ate of the produce of the land. the Manna ceased. No longer was their Manna for the Israelites, who that year ate of the yield of the land of Canaan...

Comment: Okay no more Manna, they now have corn in its stead (Tortillas, for every body)...

Ezekial 4:9

(KJV) Take then, also unto thee wheat, barley, beans, lentils, millet, fitches and put them in one vessel and make bread...

(GN) Now, take some wheat, barley, beans, peas, millet, spelt; mix them together and make bread...

(ASB) And you take wheat, barley, beans and lentils, millet and splet, and put them in a single vessel and make bread of them...

(ACB) Again, take wheat and barley and beans and lentils and millet and spelt, put them in a vessel and make bread out of them...

Comment: Here we have a mish-mash of ingredients, at a meager attempt to reproduce a heaven sent product (I wonder if god trademarked - Manna???).

Daniel 1:12 15 & 17

(KJV) Prove thy servants, I beseech thee, ten days and let them give us pulse to eat and water to drink. And at the end of the ten days their countainances appeared fairer and fatter in flesh then all the children which did eat the portion of the kings meat.....And for these four children, God gave them knowledge and skill in all learning and wisdom, and Daniel had understandings in all visions and dreams...

(GN) "Test us for ten days", he said, "give us vegetables to eat and water to drink"...When the time was up, they looked healthier and stronger, than all those who had eaten of the royal feast...God gave the four young men knowledge and skills in literature and philosophy. In addition he gave Daniel skill in interpeting dreams and visions...

(ASB) Test your servants for ten days, let us be given vegetables to eat and water to drink... And at the end of the ten days, it was seen that they were better in appearance and fatter in flesh. than all the youths who ate the king's rich food... As for this four youths, God gave them learning and skill in all letters and wisdom, and Daniel had understanding ian all vissions and dreams...

(ACB) Please, test your servants for ten days. Give us vegetables and water to drink. Then see how we look in comparison with the other young men who eat from the royal table and treat your servants according to what you see...After ten days. they looked healthier and better fed than any of the young men who ate from the royal table...To these four young men, God gave knowledge and proficiency in all literature and science and to Daniel the understanding of all visions and dreams.

Comment: Here is a realistic application of the - Altruistic Diet; it's all Good, with Great results (Food of Champions !!!). See what a vegetarian diet can do (want to bet that the pulse was Lentils) ??? I find it interesting that in the KJV, the word children, appears, for Daniel and his friends...

NEW TESTAMENT
Mathew 4:3 & 4

(KJV) And when the tempter came to him, he said;"if thou be the son of God, command that these stones be made bread"... Man shall not live by bread alone; but by every word that proceeds out of the mouth of God...

(GN) The Devil said to him,"If you are God's son, order these stones to turn to bread"...But Jesus answered,"the scripture says, human beings can not live on bread alone"...

(ASB) And the tempter came and said to him,"if you are the son of God, command that these stones become loaves of bread"... But Jesus answered,"it is written, man shall not live by bread alone, but by every word that proceeds from the mouth of God"...

(ACB) The tempter approached and said to him,"if you are the Son of God, command that these stones become loaves of bread"...He said in reply,"it is written, that one does not live by bread alone, but by every word that comes forth from the mouth of God"...

Comment: We have here the first temptation of the Christ with Bread...Remember way back in Genisis 3:9, when humanity is told to eat Bread as a punishment ??? Jesus probably knew Bread would block his neuro-pathic transmitters; clogging up his reception and transmission. Remember, also, that at the Last Supper, Jesus offered up Bread & Wine; maybe, this is why the next day while hanging on the cross, he asked God, why He'd forsakened Him...

Luke 2:36 & 37

(KJV) And there was this one prophetess, Anna...And she was a widow of about four score and four years, which departed not from the temple, but served God with fasting and prayers, night and day...

(GN) Then there was a very old prophet, a widow named Anna...she never left the temple; day and night she worshipped God, fasting and praying...

(ASB) And there was a prophetess, named Anna...she did not depart from the temple, worshipping with fasting and prayer, night and day...

(ACB) There was also a prophetess, Anna...she never left the temple, but worshipped, night and day, with fasting and prayer...

Comment: There is a lot to be said about cleaning out the plumbing, makes for less gunk on the synapses and clearer reception...(Clairvoyance and Clairessence)...

Acts 13:2

(KJV) As they ministered in the Lord and fasted, the Holy Spirit said:...

(GN) While they were serving the Lord and fasting, the Holy Spirit said to them:...

(ASB) While they were worshipping the Lord and fasting, the Holy Spirit said:...

(ACB) While they were worshipping the Lord and fasting, yhe Holy Spirit said:...

Comments: Seeing the Holy Spirit & fasting, seemed to be linked; remember that fasting, also, puts the brain into Hypo-Glycemic shock and prone to hallucinations...HHHM-MMMM !!!

1 Corinthians 3:16

(KJV) Know ye not that ye are the temple of God and that the Spirit of God dweleth in you???

(GN) Surely, you know you are God's temple and that God's Spirit lives in you...

(ASB) Do you not know that you are God's temple and that God's spirit dwels in you...

(ACB) Do you not know that you are the temple of God and that the Spirit of God dwells in you...

Comment: A clean temple (body) makes for a crystal relationship with God...In Genisis 2:19 & 20, we have Adam & God hanging out naming all the animal, which was before the expulsion from Eden (and also before the creation of Eve - women, they's all trouble !!!)...Clean Body; Clear Psyche & Shinning Soul !!!

Galatians 4:25

(KJV) for the Hager is Mount Sinai in Arabia...

(GN) Hagar, who stands for Mount Suinai, in Arabia...

(ASB) Now Hagar is Mount Sinai, in Arabia...

(ACB) Hagar represents Sinai; a mountain in Arabia...

Comment: Unless Paul is throwing us a curve ball, looks like I was corect; Mt.Sinai (aka.,Hagar; aka.,Horeb) is in Saudi Arabia (time to change the maps & tourist trade)...

1 Timothy 4:15

(KJV) Meditate upon these things, give thyself wholly to them; that thy profiting may appear to all...

(GN) Practice these things and devote yourself to them, in order that your progress may be seen by all...

(ASB) Practice these duties, devote yourself to them; so that all may see your progress...

(ACB) Be dilligent in these matters, be absorbed in them; so that your progress may be evident to everyone...

Comment: I put this in here, to highlight the importance of thinking things through and not jump to or be persuaded by the first inferences. It took a lot of thinking and trusting in the points that were being revealed to me, which differ from the teachings I have received over the years…"The people are destroyed through a lack of knowledge"…Hosea 4:6

CHAPTER 3

IT IS WHAT IT IS !!!

"IN THE BEGINNING was the Word and the Word was with God, and the Word was God..." (John1:1-KJV)..."The word is the bird and the bird is the word"...(the Surfin Bird by the Trashmen: 1963)... "Words are the greatest source of mis-understndings"... (The Little Prince by Antione Saint Exuprey)... As I read through the different religious texts, in total. they are quite different than what one is subject to at Sunday services; if truth be known, they are filled with many anomallies, which we will explore in this chapter...

Ya-see, all texts from the major religions, have the same problems; (1) they are not written by the central figures (hence others people wrote them - the word is Psuedographic) and (2) they were written years after the central figures passed on... So, what's the Big-Deal ??? Millions upon Millions of people have lost their lives and livelihoods because of this...You could be next...

We all know that David killed Goliath-right!!! Right??? Except, we read in 2 Samuel 21:19 "and Elhanan the son of Jareaoreglm, the Bethlehemite, slew Goliath, the Gittite, the shaft of whose spear, was like a weavers beam" (ASB; ACB; GN)... Sounds pretty dang big to me... Just the King James Version says it was the cousin of Goliath...

The King James Version (by-the-way) is considered the most flawed of the bibles by bibical palentologists; which should make those Sunday Morning Media Ministers some- what unconfortable... It Get's Way Better...

Why is the Truth important ??? Because too many people -mothers; fathers; children; get hurt or killed because of lies, or I should say: White-Lies or Satan's Truths, kinda what you hear on those cable programs... You know, the ones were they are yelling your opinions to you...

Just today, two terrorists bombed the subway (not the sandwich shop), in St. Peterburg, Russia... It is 2017; and peo- ple still think like it's 1017; in this day and age people still do not comprehend what they read... Islam means to HUMBLE ones self before God...Muslim means One who HUMBLES himself before God... To Humble one's self, one must abate one's own EGO... Jihad is to be against One's own EGO... You know EGO like the Original Sin - Adam and Eve - "For God doth know that in the day ye eat thereof, then your eyes shall be openned, and ye shall be as gods, knowing good and evil", (KJV - Genesis 3:5)

It is Religions and the Religious, that set people astray; so many of whom suffered the loss of their earthly fathers, at a young age or looking for their approval, that they will spend their life searching for their Heavenly Father...Muhammid, lost his father at six years old...We no longer have mention of St, Joseph, after, the boy Jesus' visit to the temple (for his Bar-Mitz-Vah)...

Just about the whole of Mathrw 23, is Jesus warnings of the Hypocrisy of the religious authorities... From the very beginning, when people began huddling in caves or gather- ing in tribes; there was always some one who sought to take advantage of them by manipulating their fears... The tribe's witch-doctor or shaman was always well taken care of for doing the least work...How many of the virgins, do you actually think were still virgins when they were sacrificed; especially after the shaman visited them...We now know, because of **PBS**, that many of the child sacrifices were to satisfy times of famine; but, of course, the children of the rulling families did not make the menu-de-jour...

Well, the Leavites turned it into professional larceny; because they stood with Moses; in Numbers Chapter 8 we read that they are to receive a tithe of all of Israel instead of land.. Wow, what a deal !!! So, now let's get into some of the jucier tid-bits... Yous probably won't be the same after this E X C U L P A T I O N !!!

Let's see, where to begin ??? How's about a real eye-popper; ahey ???

Mark 14: 50, 51 & 52 -(KJV, GN, ASB, ACB - they all read the same)...

"Then all the disciples left him and ran away. A certain young man, dressed only in a linen cloth, was following Jesus. They tried to arrest him, but he ran away naked, leaving the cloth behind."

Now don't that beat all...Jesus might have ALSO been a Homo-Sexual - I don't know, I wasn't there; but here he is, knowing he is to be arrested this evening and all the Apostles high-tail it and here is this (un-named) young man who sticks it out with him, until the authorities lay hands on him (who just happens to run away - Naked)...Sounds like a Very Special Relationship; more special than Jesus had with his Apostles... I'll bet; them HOMO-PHOBIC Ministers love this verse (and this is why we never hear this verse read in church). Now I have read pieces where the author tries to explain this away as Jesus baptizing or initiating (???) this young man. NO-where else does Jesus baptize or initiate anyone. It's all what you want to believe - especially if yous don't know your bible... The only thing that comes close is in John 20:22 -"Then Jesus breathed on them (the Apostles) and said; receive the Holy Spirit"; which kinda nullifies Pentecostal Sunday and it was also after Jesus was resurrected...

I say. ALSO, because in the -"lost Gospel of Phillip"; page 61: plate 107 - we read:..."Miriam of Mag dala, known as his companion; for him Miriam is a sister, a mother and a wife"... and in Phillip, logion 55:3-4; we read -"The Teacher loved her (Miriam) more than all the disciples, he often kissed her on the mouth"...And this was in the days before mouth-wash...

Yous remember: "Mary (or Miriam, for the Hebrews) Mag dala. from whom Jesus had driven out seven demons." (Mark 16:9) and I'm assuming he did this before he kissed her on the mouth... Mary Mag dala was known as Jesus' consort, which means she shared in convivial privilages (maybe that DaVinci code story wasn't so far off of the mark)...In "the Gospel of Mary of Magdala" we read in PRyl 463 - "If the Savior considered her worthy, who are you to disregard her. For he knew her completely and loved her steadfastly...Geee; I wonder what else the church kept out of the Conical Bible - we will get to that in a future chapter.

Here's another one I like, it has to do with money - Yous may like it, also...In Acts chapter 5: we read the story of Ananias and Sapphira, who vowed to sell all they had and give it all to the Apostles -(SWEET)-, but decided to keep some for a rainy day; in 4-5 we read:"...You have not lied to people, but to God. As soon as Ananias heard this he fell down dead." This is after the end of Acts chapter 4 were others, like Barnabas, had sold every thing they owned and gave it to the Apostles. (Ya see he bought his way in.) Where else, other than religions, can you get people to sell their everything and hand the MULA over (Remember this is in the days before social progtams and most probably why Saul re-invented himself as Paul)...

Money has a lot to do with all the mess we expeience !!! "You can not serve both God and money." (Mathew 6:24)... Isn't it amazing how the religious work us over to give up as much, even all of our worth. We are suppose to have faith that God will provide; but the religious miser all the donations away in bank acounts and holdings. What a Great-Scam !!! With hurricain Harvey damaging a large section of Texas & the Gulf area, many people are agoog, still, that a Monied Millionaire Media Minister did not open his Arena/House of Worship to those in NEED of shelter & comfort...Doesn't make me wonder a bit...

We are suppose to do alot with less, while the religious, move into multi-million dollar mansions; live in villas on the Gulf with their own air-strip and hanger with multipule planes; have no shame in asking their flock for donations of sixty million dollars to purchase a new private plane, so's they can travel with their entourage; spend forty million dollars to upgrade their villa in Austria and my personal favorite; spend 500 million dollars (this would purchase a lot of bowels of musch) , to built a citadel on a mountain top, which they just happen to own the mountain and continue to purchase more of it and last but not least, estimated net worth of three quarters (3/4) of a Billion Dollars (and this person is as dry as sawdust)... Who says; getting closer to God doesn't have its perks ???

I was fortunate to witness Media Ministers bragging (I believe it's called "Willy-Wagging"), on how the government better not touch THEIR MONEY, because that very same government has taught them to kill with their hands. (Ain't it wonderful how our donations, become THEIR MONEY $$$). One of my favorites is, when a minister mentioned - how the religions were "persecuted" in 2004 when the government, called them all in to explain; What they were actually doing with the Donations, making their tax-exempt status conditional on their disbursemnet of funds to charities. TAX-EXEMPT STATUS ??? Where in the Constitution does it grant them a tax-exempt status ??? There is the -"Freedom of Religion" ; along with the Press: but no freedom from paying taxes. Hence the pillferring continues. Keeping in mind ROMANS 13:6-"That is why you should also pay taxes: because the authorities are working for God when they fulfill their duties." ('m guesing. this one doesn't mean what it says, either !!!)

We should be well aware that religion is all about money... The Protestant Reformation was started by Martin Luther because he did not want to pay his tithes to the Vatican. He nailed his grievences (he was being easy on them, because I am no fan of what the Church has done to people over these two milleniums) on the door of the local church and by the time he returned to his little nouck of the planet; seeing what the people had done; he repented of his action. He them married an ex-nun, with whom he had six children (I'm guessing this acted as a distraction or penance; depending how you look at it)...

Now, it is interesting to me that these Protestants call themselves -"people of the word"; especially when it is convenient for them. It is these same -"people of the word", who gloss over Mathew 16:16-19-"Simon Peter answered, "You are the the Messiah, the Son of God" "Good for you, Simon, son of John,: Jesus answered, "For this truth did not come to you from some human being, but it was given to you directly by my Father (Da Big Ka-Who-Na, Himself, picked Peter, VERY INTERESTING)...And so I tell you, Peter, you are a rock and on this rock foundation I will build my church and not even death will be able to over come it...I will give you the keys to the Kingdom of Heaven; what you porhibit on earth, will be porhibited in heaven; what you permit on earth will be permitted in heaven"...(GN)

It is amazing to me how much Martin Luther got WRONG !!! He said that Jesus instituted the sacraments of Baptism and Marriage; NO-NO-NO; Jesus participated in these along with Confirmation or Bar-Mitz-Vah for the Hebrews (Luke 2:41 & 42), where the boy Jesus is in the temple (this, by the way, is the last time we hear mention of St.Joseph)...Jesus did institute the Sacraments of Penance (which I've cited in the previous paragrah); Eucharist (which was the Last Supper) ; Holy Orders (which I've cited John 20:22 and Anointing of the Sick (Mark 14:3-9)...

Martin Luther, also, came up with the notion of the "Gospel of Grace" (maybe because he plagued himself with guilt over some sin ???), which tells us - God forgives... Yes but God Does NOT Forget; Like God did not forget the sin of Adam & Eve and Condemed humanity with it, which is at the Alpha (or beginning) of the Bible and in Revelation 20:12, the Omega (or end) of the Bible, we read -"and another book was opened, which is the book of life and the dead were judged out of those things which were written in the books, according to their works". Looks like to me that God Ain't a Forgettin !!!

When it comes to Sickness - we read in James 5:14 -"Are any among you sick? They should send for the church elders who will pray for them and rub olive oil on them, in the name of the Lord"; where these Monied-Ministers and families, go to the best doctors, clinics and hospitals, around this world, for their treatments; some have even been resurrected so they can continue with their assignment; while the rest of us have to contend with feeling like a salad...

This is just some of the stuff I found in the New testament; now let us turn our attention to the Old Testament (when the foundation is tilted, so goes the structure - look at the Tower of Pisa)...There are quite a few good books, written by bibical palenthologists (those who check this stuff out with a fine tooth comb); and they all agree that most of the Old Testament or Hebrew Torah are stories, expounded upon by the Hebrews, taken from the Egyptian, Bablyonian and some Greek mythology; (for example the story of Ester and the feast of Purim was a Babylonian festival, brought back by the Hebtews, after they returned from captivity). The story of Samson. is just the Hebrews plagarizing of the Greek's story of Hercules.

I have already mentioned the story of Elhanan and Goliath; how's about, according to the Bible Adam and Eve were the first Hebrews not the first man and woman...We pick up the story of creation on the sixth day- Genesis 1: 27 -"so God created man in his image, in the image of God created he him: male and female created he them" (KJV)... This is a double wammy; first off, God did not create Adam until Genesis 2:7, after the seventh day-also known as the day of rest and yous can be more convinced of this when you read the chronology of the generations ; and by the way this also tidies up the Cain and Seth, who were left over, after the murder of Abel having children with their Mom-Eve; (although incest would explain, why humanity is all screwed up)...

Second, and I really like this for the Homo-Phobic Ministers -God is Trans-Gender, Bi-Sexual, Hermaphrodite, Inter-Sexual (is the updated terminology); what ever term yous like... No-No-No, that's not what it means; oh yeah, that's what it says - Ye People of the Word; "male and female created he them -in his image."

Actually Eve wasn't even the first female-Hebrew; it was Lilith, according to the Hebrew Torah she was created with Adam and was equal to him (how's bout them apples woman suffergets). When we read the more common story, God creates Adam, breathing life into him; hence rendering him, his soul and Eve is just plopped there. This gives rise to Plato's Split-Soul Theory.

Heck, if you go back and read the fifth and sixth day of creation in Genesis (slowly, with comprehension); it is very similar to Charles Darwin's - Theory of Evolution - in the "Origen of the Species" (what a con-ink-i-dent; Hey)... So, why are the religious still at odds with science ??? Answer : Money !!! In Isaiah 40:22 we read -"It is He that sitteth upon the circle of the earth, and the inhabitants thereof are as grasshoppers; that stretcheth out the heavens as a curtain and spreadeth them out as a tent to dwell." In modern day physics, we have confirmation that the universe is EXPANDING, some say from the initial Energy of the - Big Bang, (which was a theory initiated by a friar working in the Vatican's Dept. of Sciences in the 1600's) into Multi-Verses !!!

When yous look at the bible in it's entirety; God does not come out looking to good...He starts out by creating the Heavenly Host and on the top of his list is the Arch-Angel Samel, (whom the Greeks term Satan- the deceiver or in Latin- Lucifer the bearer of light)...God gussies him up, inflating his ego and when he hears that God has another great idea, of creating humanity, Samel losses it and defects with a large number of the heavenly host... So; How Good can Heaven Really Be ???

Not learning his leason, (Remember : Parents - DO NOT SPOIL YOUR CHILDREN; it never turns out well) God proceeds to give Adam everything, even a main squeeze (I'm guessing them sheep weren't enough on a cold night; BBBAAAAA)...Loe and behold; Samel appears (bearing light on the situation) and shows humanity for what they are - EGOTISTS (Genesis 1:26 -"And God said: let us make man in our image, after our likeness..." It is the LIKENESS part, that's the sinker for humanity; because God is a BIG-EGOTIST (according to the Bible)...

That doesn't go well, so he throws them out of Eden and curses humanity to hard labor. God is so fed up with human-ity, that by Genisis 6:5 - "God repented from the creation of humanity'...Do you know what it takes for God to REPENT ??? So He brings about the Great Flood and washes away his iniquity, along with most all of life, hoping for a fresh start... Not- with-standing, this doesn't work, so God decides to come up with some rules and calls them COMMANDMENTS, ten (10) to be precise...Which no-one pays any attention to; let me just focus on the fifth-"Thou shalt not kill", which all the religions have violated. In Exodus 20; God gives the Hebrews these Ten Commandments and by Numbers 15:32-38, we read the story of a man, "who God says to be put to death because he was collecting firewood on the Sabbath..." God must have a case of the FOGOTTS. Just think if the religous institutions focused on not lying or not commiting adultery - THE SEATS WOULD BE EMPTY !!!

Maybe, God is Bi-Polar...In Genesis 9:6, after the Great Flood, we read-"whoso sheddeth man's blood, by man shall his blood be shed..."; but in Genesis 4:15, we see God put a sign on Cain's forehead, so no one is to harm him. Looks like God was feeling a little guilty; maybe he MIS-Communicated with Cain and Abel, about thier sacrifices...Remeber Cain brought vegetation form the fields and God said not good enough - I like me some bar-be-que and Abel's lamb looks so juicy...Actually, the vegetation is for human consumption; is probably what He meant to say (Pho-Pa)...

Well, I've digressed; so the laws don't work out well, so God decides to send his only begotten Son...(Did yous know, that because of the lineage that is given to us in Mathew 1; Jesus is either the son of God or the Messiah, but can not be both. To be the Messiah one had to be of the lineage from David, from Abraham, from Adam; well the lineage goes to Joseph. Jesus was begotten of the Holy Spirit which means Jesus could not be the Messiah; for Jesus to be the Messiah, it means that Joseph had to be getting him some. Mary is not mentioned in any lineage, even though we assume she is Hebrew and there are no adoptions allowed (yous know them Eugenisists theys need to tie presumed authority to the past); so it's male begets male begets male, etcetera...So Jesus comes to die for our sins (which we didn't even commit; but really placates our EGO)... Makes us feel special !!!

This doesn't work out so well, because we read in Revelations (by the way; probably written by a second century monk named Certinius) that everything is going to HECK in a hand-basket...Then Jesus is coming back, after everyone is KAPUT, to set up God's kingdom on earth...Why ??? Nothing has worked out correctly, Yet !!! All this lead a second century bishop - Marcineas - to hypothesis, that there must be three (3) gods: the Creator God, the Evil God and the family idiot god, whom they put in charge of overseeing the business here on earth...Even though, in light of everything, this makes sense, it got Marcineas ex-communicated...Oh well, that's the way the hypothesis crumbles...

So, if the Bible is so flawed, Why have I put yous through this ??? Because, it still is a good source of recipes for one's daily traumas and because, it reads like a great novel, with all that passion & pain and because, it is a good study in sociology (human behavior) and because, in the next few chapters I will be leading yous through what I had to go through, just to get to the truth of lentils being Manna...

Quite an ordeal to come to know the Truth...So, how are yous enjoying the scanvenger hunt so far ???

C H A P T E R 4

MOZARELLA

THAT BUTTERY SOFT milky cheese mounds, still warm, in its own water, partnered with a fresh vine rippened tomato from the garden; equal-sliced rounds laid on a platter, lightly sprinkled with pinches of salt and oregano, with drizzles of qualtiy pure extra virgen olive oil, accompanied by a finely hand made and baked loaf of Italian bread with a crisp crust and nicely air pocketed interior and one would insult this dish without a fine bottle of red frizcante or sangiovese wine... HHMM; stick me with a fork, cause I'm done.

I just wanted to give yous a mental image, that would make you salivate (good thing Jesus wasn't Italian, cause I doubt he'd be able to fast for 40 days if he was)... I wanted to get to the Italian verb - MOZZATA; che vo dire ; which, in english, means to pull apart (like American taffy), which is what we are to embark on here.

As part of our continuing scavenger-hunt, we are going to get our hands into the history of the Old Testament, the New Testament and the written word; so's we can make some rational sense of the passages in Chapter 2...We are going to let our minds, pull apart and then re-fashion it all into pallatable mounds of digestive delight for our heads,(hence, the visual imagery at the beginning of this chapter...

47

Where to Start ??? Let us begin with the written word this will aid us in bringing these parts together (Like the hot water that we begin the Mozzarella process)...The Old Testament or Torah, we will consider the milk, that nurtures and the New Testament as the renin or acid that makes the milk curdle and solidify, so once placed in the hot water, causing the protiens to relax enough so one may form balls, mounds, braids or whatever(yous can tell I've done this before).

The written word, as we know it today - letters, that make up definable words, words that make up comprehendible sentences, sentences that make up purposeful paragraphs, paragraphs that make up knowlege filled chapters, chapters that make up theme filled works that present hypothisis and theories, that are supported or not by those words; (wow, what a mouth full); came about approximately in 1,000 A.D. (Anno Domini) or about 1,000 years ago, give or take a few centuries...

So, the form you are reading at present, has only been around for about 1,000 years; which was transcribed by hand until 1439, with the invention of the Guttenberg Press... What was before that ??? A hieroglyphics system were symbols were used to represent words and the only ones who knew how to decifer it were the scribes that wrote and INVENTED IT. The system of writting we enjoy today, developed through a cumbersome process...

The scribe was the most important person at the kings court, He was the only one who knew what he wrote and could change the meanings, depending on the situation. (Just think, if the scribe developed dementia; what a mess.)...Keep in mind, that the wholesale educating of the masses has only been with us for maybe the past 100 years, definately since the 1,930's... Education was for the wealthy or well to do...

Why, Heck, Andrew Carneige, as a poor youngin was not allowed into libraries; so's when he became a BILLIONAIRE in 1901 (not that was real money) funded libraries for the general public...(Interesting how memory is selective; he remembered the library incident, but forgot the poverty part, keeping his workers impoverished through his adult life.)

Have you ever used Roman Numerals ??? Certain letters have numerical values and the sum worth would depend upon the positioning of those letters. Letters of a lesser numerical value placed infront of those of greater value, would lessen the sum total. Such as M = 1,000 and L = 50; so MLM = 1950 and MML would = 2050. Symbols placed before meant one thing and something else if placed after (what a mis-mash)...

Now, let's use your "Little Grey Cells" and envision that all the words yous are reading are acually symbols, without spacing, without punctuation, without paragraphs - have you got the picture. UGH !!! Think of trying to read oriental symbols (I believe, there are 232) from top to bottom, without knowing what they meant or even better (for that rubics cube mind bender) having a rudimentry knowledge of them symbols' meaning...Is Your Head Pounding, Yet???

I have taken issue with this because the Hebrews did not have a written language before Moses; raised in the house of Pharoh, as a Prince of Egypt, lead them out of Egypt and wandering about (probably looking for a good all-night Diner)... Remember, the Hebrews were slaves or servants (which ever term yous prefer), whom de-fin-a-tive-ly were not educated. Faced with nation building, Moses and his inner circle, had need to delineate and place things in some sort of order and using dried animal skins, for paper, and dried fruit juice attempted to put something together.

Developing a written language is the foundation of any government. Ya just can't tell peoples nothin, cause theys got an attention span like the life time of a G-nat. Now Moses and his marauders go about developing a language; like the Egyptians, whom, they just departed from and all the other nations of their time.

The Hebrews were very good plagarists; they plagarized the Egyptians for stories and a written language, developing their own symbols for words -(keep in mind that the scribes knew the key of the language: VERY IMPORTANT). And got a Big-Ass Bodyguard to enforce it - GOD !!!

Why do I bring this up ??? Ah, what I have been describing till now is the first half of the Old Testament. Aproximately 1,000 years after Moses comes Ezra, whom is approximately 350 years before Jesus. Here, the Hebrews also plagarized the Bablyonians and Greeks (because Alexader - the Great ??? had already fashioned a highway throught this region to India) , in their 100 years of captivity, for stories. A great deal happened in this time frame.

As the story goes (and there seems to be no end to stories); as the Babylonians are escorting the Upper Crust Hebrews out of Jerusalem (city of peace ???), they take with them anything and everything they can get there hands on. In this 100 year time frame, Ezra and his Rabbis come across Moses' writtings that were in the temple. (Ya gotta wonder what they were doing before this ???) They now set about to develop the Torah (you know, those two hug scrolls, they carry in front of them)...

Try using your imagination for this - the Hebrews are in exile, they come across dried animal skins with writting on them, which was from a thosand years before. How much of this do you think was -Legible ??? How much of this do you think they embelished or Fudged (to use a modern colloquilism; which is worth 4 bitts)??? I seemed to have noticed that they have problems with numbers; to me they seem embellished (or greatly exaggerated, to use the vernacular)... Aproximately, half way throught he Old Testament we come to the stories of Ezra and Nathaniel, were this is made evident and all the stories afterwards are juxtaposed loosing their timeline, from the Hebrews period of captivity in Babylon.

It is a little alarming, when you consider that people are bringing about - End of the World - scenarios from these stories; that will now lead us to the New Testament. I have already mentioned some lost Gospels and some Canonical Gospels, which share the same thing - they are PSEUDEPIGRAPHIC (now there's a 3 dollar word for yous), which means, written by some one other than. As is the Koran, whom Muhammid also plagarized stories from the Hebrew and Christian sects that habitated his region of Mecca, which was very pagan at the time...

The Old Testament has these Blatant-Glaring problems, which now proliferates into the New Testament and even the Koran. When the foundation of a building (or religion) is askew then, as the work progresses it is in danger of collapsing (think of the tower of Pisa). There is little wonder as to why this world is ready to explode, because of these religions. The Muslims are in a conundrum : to rightfully deny the Hebrews their patch in Palestine is to also deny the root of their own religion.

Let us stroll through a historical synopsis of the New Testament, the reason being that - I want to and that some passages bring light to bear upon my thesis. Okay; Jesus dies and the Apostles are scattered. The Resurrection gives them a renewed hope, but they are still worried about their own necks. The Holy Spirit pays them a visit on Pentecostal Sunday (which, by the way, is a Hebrew holiday) and they are enboldened.

"They were all filled with the Holy Spirit and began to talk in other languages, as the Spirit enabled them to speak." (Acts 2:4)..."How is it, then. that all of us hear them speaking in our own native languages." (Acts 4:8)...So all these ministers babbling in, in-com-pre-hen-sible jibberish is just that; for shock-n-awe of the simple minded.

Now all the Apostles go about the business of starting a new religion; Peter and Paul end up in Rome (if Mary had joined them, they probably could of rocked the Vatican, way back when)... It takes approximately 300 years and the insistance of the then Roman Emperor Constantine, to force - The Church - to put something together. The Council of Nicea is convenied in 324 A.D. where - The Church - begins the process of putting writtings to paper. It is not till 1624 A, D. when the Council of Trent is convenied to solidify, what we now know today as "Da Bible".

Keep the following in mind: Jesus and his Dusty-Dozen, where for all intent purposes ILLITERATE (you would think Da-Big-Guy would send people who could write, being that He wanted to convey a message)...Mathew, maybe, had rudimentary literacy, being that he was a tax collector. In the beginning of the Gospel of Mathew we are presented with a run down of the Hebrew lineage for the Messiah; starting from Adam down to Joseph (which is a lot shorter than that presented to us in the Old Testament). In this lineage there are no adoptions and no females; so Jesus, is either the Son of God or the Messiah; he can not be both (according to the Bible)....Let's not forget that Luke, was supposedly a doctor and paired with Paul and that Mark paired with Peter...

If yous remember way back at the beginning of this chapter, I walked us through the history of the written word. Jesus and his gang spoke in Arimaeic (which the Koran is written in)... Others, 60 to 120 years later wrote down what was told to them by intermediaries, can you remember conversations you had 60 years ago??? Written in what ever language of the time, maybe into Greek, then maybe Roman. then into Greek or Egyptian, then maybe into Latin and eventually into indiginous languages, like English (giving the term - lost in translation its UMPH).

The Koran also suffers from this malady of Convenient Memory and is also, psuedographic, because they did not start writting it till 20 years after Muhammid passed on, not to mention that most all of the correlated references to the Old & New Testaments, were picked up by Muhammid (the messenger, according to the Koran) while traveling with his uncle (who adopted him because his mother died, just after his birth and his father died when he was six years old) from the time he was seven (7) years old and the Hebrew & Christian tribes that habitated his region at the time and conveniently (or through lack of remembering) or by being inventive changed some of the specifics of the stories, to make them his own... Muslims celebrate a holiday based on a dream, Muhammid had, of the story of Abraham & Issach, re-inventing the detalis...

The Bible was the first book to be printed on the Guttenberg press, until then things were copied by hand by cloistered members of the clergy (they were the educators of the times). Bibical palenthologists have spent their lives, track-ing down the earliest copies of bibles. These copies show how the transcribers missed parts, made mistakes, edited, added to, altered and any other human contrivance immaginable, copied by succeeding generations...

The disciple Luke was supposedly a doctor, hence some-what literate and the adjatent to Saul, the rabbi from Trasus. Luke is accredited with the Gospel of Luke and Acts and helping Paul with his letters, especially references Paul makes to Jesus' ministry, since Paul was not part of the inner circle. Also, not written by Luke...

The Episcles of Paul (which Martin Luther, conveiently used to split The Church) are the earliest pieces included in The Bible. Letters written by a person who had no direct contact with Jesus, whose frist mention was "holding cloakes of the Elders as they stoned Stephen to death (Acts 7:57)... and Saul approved of the murder." (Acts 8:1)...Paul, who is pestered by a demon; ..."there was given to me a thorn in the flesh, the messenger of Satan to buffet me." (2 Corinthians 12:7), Paul who tells us that "Even Satan (which is Greek for -the deceiver) can disguise himself to look like an angel of light" (2 Corinthians 11:14); Paul who was converted on the road to Damascus, while ridding on a donkey, by a flash of light (Acts 9:3-7); Paul whom I consider; a tool of Grand Deception to Christianity...

Just this morning, after Cookie got me up early for her walk, I settled down to watch one of these Media Ministers' progam, where-in, he states; that the Four (4) Canonical Gospels, along with the works of Peter, James & John (you know, Jesus' lead-off hitters) are "Satanic-Deceptions" and that the writtings of Paul (aka., Saul) are the True Christian Gospel...This is the same minister that gets all excited & gidy over Revelation and the Rapture, that he believes he will part of...Not to burst his bubble, but, Saint John the Divine, was supposed to have authored Revelations, the same one that he accuses of "Satanic-Deceptions"...It is a good thing that his viewers do not have a good memory...

Two (2) days after this, after another early morning walk with Cookie; I am watching another Millionare Media Minister or I should say - reading, (because I use the - closed caption when the air conditioning is running, LESS NOISE, (there is enough noise in the world) and every time this specific minister speaks of Satan or Demons, the letters get so scrambled up into an incomprehensible language, kinda like, when one plays a record back-wards.. I guess them Pixies were working overtime...Very Interesting !!!

Being that I have strayed to this topic, the story goes that Muhammid (a misogynystic, philandering, pedophile, his second wife, his favorite, being six (6) years old, he being 50 years old), while in the cave he frequented (because his first wife, whom mysteriouly died after conversion to Islam, was fed up with him throwing him out of the tent to go sleep with the camels), being cold & hungry (probably left without lunch) was seized by the Arch-Angel Gabriel (the messenger) by the throat and told to recite...Now don't that beat all; through out scripture, it is NOT the angels of God that attack humans. Also, a story relayed by one of those morning ministers, that while cleaning out a specific structure was choked, by the throat, by some demon and goes on to say that they are all - Blow & No Go; so I'm guessing it was his imagination that was choking him ???

This shows a tremndous amount of ambiquity for something that is to be - the Absolut Word of God...(The old Bar-Tender adage is true - Believe none of what you HEAR & half of what you SEE)...I have stated, previously, that for lies to be successful, there must be present a grain (or seed, in our case) of truth...

There has been that, some thing, that has been tugging at the coat-tails of humanity ever since the beginning, desperately needing to be heard. Hence, is why in John 8:32, Jesus admonishes us - "and ye shall know the truth (which has been no easy task) for the truth shall set you free"... What about the Seeking - the Journey (if yous will) ??? There's a wrinkle for your krinkle !!! Jesus probably surmised that the Truth & Love, are one in the same...

C H A P T E R 5

THE WAY

AFTER JESUS'S DEATH and resurrection, for a few centuries the Apostles, disciples and later Christians were termed - followers of the way - which terminology we see in Acts...We are not going to follow that way here; but the way something, like Bread, enters and then exits, through our bodies...(this'll be some interesting STUFF)...

Most people are use to gobbling down some chow and - Presto Changeo - a plop, splash and flush away, no one gives it another thought; unless, that is, that things don't turn out the way it should. Then its laxatives or fiber or a trip to the proctologists office. After a visit to the dentist office, one usually gets a lolly; what does one get after a visit to the proctologists office ? Your guess is as good as mine...

It is no mistake that the illnesses of today are considered the - "Diseases of the Wealthy"... Maybe, that's why in Mathew 19:24, Jesus admonishes us with - "it is easier for a camel to go through the eye of a needle, than for a rich man to enter into the kingdom of God". The first new thing on the market is usually expensive, because of a low unknown market share. So the wealthy gobble it up (literally), because they can afford to pay...

Take raw cane sugar, for instance. When Chris Columbus brought it back to Spain, from one of his (5) island ventures (this is why Columbus never discovered the New World; but did establish the first tour excurrsions to the Carribean), the wealth of society, from the crown to all around, could not get enough of it. Then the illnesses started, like - Diabetes (aka., wasting disease); added to the breads the people were already ingesting, became a perfect storm for the human body...Peolpe could not get enough of sugar, so it spread to the other nations; and so did disease !!!

Let's take a look (figuratively) at what happens to Bread as it takes its trip through our self... First off, Bread starts off as a grain. Humans do not have the enzymes to digest grains. The grain is pulverized into a dust, we call flour, add some water and yeast and we have some gloppy stuff, that we will place in an oven and magic happens; a loaf of crunchy, golden brown, warm nurturing piece of heaven emerges, whose aroma fills ones senses making the knees weak and the mouth salivate. In Old England, they would mix in hot water to the flour, called it - gruel - and ate it, making paste for their intestines... This is probably why Scrooge was so miserable...

In that saliva are the enzymes that will begin the attempt to digest that Bread. After mastication (get your minds out of the gutter), chewing the Bread, it slides down into the stomach (or tummy, for we simple people), were acids begin to break it down and muscles churn it about. The stomach also needs blood to facilitate the digestion, drawing blood from other parts of the body. The bigger the meal, the bigger the drawing of blood and this is why many are told not to go swimming or why the sand-man visits after a meal...

It then passes it onto the Small intestine, where peristalsis, the muscles that keeps every thing moving, takes over, to keep things-a-movin. The pancreas, begins to releases insulin, a hormone, to digest the Bread and bile enters the picture to help out. In the small intestine vitamins and minerals are absorbed; so if a piece of Bread is not digested, then the residue can stick to the walls, creating build-up, blocking further absorption of nutrition. Think of a lifetime of this ???

Some, may be broken down enough to get pushed through the walls, Then what ? This residue creates build up through the body...Think of a house that has never been dusted; the build up becomes noticeable in the attic, or brain as dementia; about the glands and organs, creating dysfunction and missed signals; in the joints, creating arthrtis; to our skin, the largest organ of our body, blocking pores, so wastes can not exscape and sun can not activate our Vitamin D; through out the body causing most all of the preventable infirmaries humanity suffers today. Eccetera - Eccetera - Eccetera...

To much build up in the body creates AIDS (Auto Immune Deficency Syndrome), where there is so much stuff in the body that the Immune System is constantly on the offensive, wearing itself down and missing the true invaders, causing a pandemic, like Influenza in 1918 affecting over 500 million people and Cancer today...My dog, Chelsea was diagnosed with AIDS; she subsisted on a processed dog-food diet...I changed her diet to cooked meats and some vegetables and the next year - NO AIDS !!!

I began thinking of Diabetes, in this way, when our local pharmacist, a man from India, a Vegetarian his whole life, some one in good shape, told me he had Diabetes. Of course it was easy for him to get medicine for this, but got me Ta-Thinking differently about these illnesses that we have now come to consider common. If yous watch the commericial, where they show these obviously obese people and the caption reads (reading is fundamental)," one third (1/3) of the people suffering from Diabetes are over-wiegth or obese"... Which also means; that two thirds (2/3) of the people suffering from Diabetes - ARE NOT - over wieght or obese...Hence, is why I have stated that BREAD, as a filler, is the mistake Vegetarians & Vegans, and all of us, make !!!

Diabetes (aka., Wasting Disease) results, when the pancreas is constantly pumping out insulin to digest foods, aka., excess sugar in the body, to the point that it wears itself out and then you need to take insulin (a hormone). Without insulin to digest foods; these foods would rot and become putrid through out our system. I have just previously mentioned that Diabetes is also known as (aka.,) the - Wasting Disease...

I make mention, within this book, that human beings DO NOT have the enzymes to digest grains. Inflamation in the joints and the deterioration of the cartilage that acts as cushioning for them joints, are another by product of this. My aunt suffered from deterioration of those cushions or discs, in her spine. She became the perfect storm for the MERSA Virus, which them morfed into the CANCER Virus. I still remember advising her two (2) years earlier to give up her cereal each morning. She finally got fed up and retorted - "I can't live without cereal"!!! She was correct...

It is interesting (to me, at least) that cats do not have the enzymes to digest a fresh kill; this is why cats will catch their prey, bat it around (instesd of sinking their teeth into it) till it dies, let it sit some time and begin to putrify, so as to allow the prey's own enzymes to commence the digestion process for them and answers the Quandery of one Millionare Media Minister, who happened to notice this act while camping (and why I read more than one book)...

Two (2) months before my Chelsea passed away (on July 2,2017; during the writing of this book), the vet took x-rays of her spine, because I was searching for the reason her rear right leg was weak. We found that her spine was fusing, which, like my aunt, means that the discs or cushions, had degenerated. I am well aware of Aqua Puncture Injections, which I had also explained to my aunt, before her ordeal commenced. Like my aunt, my Chelsea, because of a lapse of the vet, did not make it...

We now go into the Large Intestine, after our little diversions, which is kinda like the sewage plant of the body. Water is absorbed here and the rest is packaged for shippment to the Egress. All Done !!!

What about dairy products, like milk or cheese ??? Ever since I was a kid, I loved Cappucino, steamed-frothy milk with a shot of espresso. When Mom would take me with her, for whatever, and she stopped for an espresso, you guessed it, I got a cappucino (this was my treat). Then later in life, when I took Mom out for an espresso, I treated myself to a cappucino. After Mom & Pops passed on, I would go out, every day, to have my cappucino, as a homage & because I liked it. Well, for many a year now, every morning my sinuses would be clogged and I would easily go through a box of tissues per week. I recently stopped having a cappucino and I now go through a box of tissues per month.

My cousin, the one that ate himself to death; he was so full of Krap (literally) that his skin was greenish and no one in his family cared enough to notice...The final diagnosis was that he had a over-abundance or build-up of CO2 - Carbon Dioxide in his body. He was constantly blowing his nose, with very little result. All the Breads, Pasta, Cheeses, Cakes and what-ever-else, he was shoving in his mouth, had built up to a critical level and very probably, settled in his lungs & sinuses, so the exchange of gases - oxygen to carbon dioxide - was impeded; hence is why he'd fall asleep while sitting in a chair. His family (they's tink they's - Da SHMAT ones) would make fun of him, then shove a bowl of pasta in front of him, watch him eat it, then slowly fall asleep in the bowl in front of him - Stupid is; as Stupid does !!!

Starches also create this milky stuff that clogs us up; if yous will remember back to Chapter (1) One, when I spoke of washing rice...If you were to leave dried pasta, from the box, in a bowl of water, for some time, yous would notice that it would turn into a bowl of musch (or gruel is what the Dickins story portarys Mr. Scrooge as eating)...Hence, sprouting grains & legumes is preferrable to the human system !!!

Well, the voyage is pretty much the same, except for some variations. The important thing with diary is to remember that humans begin loosing the enzymes to digest dairy at six (6) months of age; hence is why we have many a Lactose intolerant adults. As dairy journeys through our system, its deposts mucos, as grain does, but seems to, more so, localize in the head and repiratory systems.

In the first chapter, I mentioned how Chelsea and myself suffered disorientation after a month of goat's milk. It was probably affecting our inner ear balance. Also, the sinuses become clogged. When one can not breath correctly, the brain becomes oxygen deprived and enters into a - State of Stress.. Ears, Nose and Throat are a connected system...

What happens when our bodies are stressed ??? We become more stressed; we can't breath correctly; we eat more sugars to compensate; we don't think correctly, listening to those voices in our heads as they become more virtulent. In other words we enter into a down- ward spiral of degeneration.

We all Love Meat ??? Actually. it seems to have been an after-thought on the Big-Guy's part. If you remember back in Chapter # 2; in the Genesis 9:3 account; after the Great-Flood, God gives the people his Okie-Dokie to eat meats... What happened; did Noah & his clan jump the gun and bar-be-que on board. To be fair; God did not let them know, how long their excursion was to be, beforehand...It is difficult to pass up a juicy steak on the Bar-Be-Que; ahey !!!

So, what happens to meat as we devour it ??? Pretty much the same process as the others; with the exception, that our bodies need more hydrochloric acid to digest meats. Thus developing a more acidic condition within our bodies, throwing off our PH balance, making us more prone to illnesses. There is also a time factor, meaning that it takes longer to digest meats; hence being in our systems longer, becoming putrid !!!

Ya-See, the human body is to be more on the alkaline side (provided by the ingestion of Vegetation, Legunes, Fruits & Nuts)...The more alkaline, the better the atmosphere for good health. Meats take longer for the body to digest, which also keeps the acids in our systems longer... In our day & age, our meat ratio is off the charts, also increasing our Omega 6 inbalance, making for an acidic environment and ripe for Cancer...

Meats, though, have some definate nutritional values and should be eaten sparingly; hence is why a SMALL amount of meat is included in the Altruistic Diet and was probably an after thought by Da Big Chef - GOD. Beef, is the only place we find B-12 and folic acid, which aids in the development of the spine and red blood cells...Carinvors, like Dogs, have an acidic system; that's why a vegetarian diet could slowly kill them...

Let us now look at the voyage of some vegetation or fruits The process is the same just the outcome (excuse the punny-pun) is more disreable. First off, Fruits, Legumes and Vegetation are BIO-AVAILABLE (a GREAT word), a very important word, for our health. Also, there is a plethora of Lean Proteins, Vitamins and Minerals for us to FEAST on. If this was not enough, the Piece-de-Resintence; it's about the FIBER.

Fiber, the stuff that Good Bowel Movements, are made of. Sweaping away the stuff in our intestines, that are just hanging around or hanging on the walls; making them glisteny clean. The cleaner our intestines, the more proficent the uptake of nutriets, the better out health... In the 1800's, the then Knig of England, had an autopsy performed on a man deemed to die at the age of 150 years; they found out of the ordinary - a clean intestine !!!

It is a very good thing that fruits are included as part of this Altruistic Diet, because they act as a natural laxative (King John of England, actually defecated to death after eating a bushel of peaches, while lost in the forest - I guess one may say he Krapped his Knickers), beneficially being paired with nuts. Nuts by themselves can be difficult to digest, getting caught in the - nooks & crannies of the intestine, caussing diverticulits. Yous probably did not know that your cell phone antenna are patterned after the intestines, which resemble broccoli florets, allowing more surface area for absorption.

If that wasn't enough, as this fiber gets into our system, the Sterols, (little fiber or scroubing bubbles) clean up our arteries and viens. De-Clogging the Gunky build-up that prevents the even flow of blood, which carries oxygen and nutrition through out our system... Literally, We Can Eat Ourselves Healthy !!! Also, remember vinegar, as you eat your salads and vegetation; the acids and revisterol are excelent cleaning crews for our arteries, over time...

A suggestion I made in my first book - "Cooking for Mom & Pops" - was to keep a diary. A simple composition book would do, that you can purchase at the local store. Draw a line down the middle of each page, place the date & day at the top and above each half write - What I ate today and How I feel today...You will notice that what you ate today will effect how you feel tomorrow and vice-a-versa, how you feel today is effected by what you ate yesterday... Ya-See, this is not brain surgery !!!

THE POWER OF NUTRITION

IN THE SPRING of 2016 the USCDC-(United States Center for Disease Control), issued a statement: 90% of Cancers is due to diet... (BAM)...I started this chapter with something that would smack you between the eyes and wake you right up,

How can they say that ??? What they don't tell you is that Cancer is a virus and one catches it like other viruses and one disposes of it like other viruses, with a healthy immune system and is encouraged and supported by a healthy diet...YEP, IT IS AS SIMPLE AS THAT...

Ya-see, our body's system is PHENOMINAL...Here's how it works (I Love This), as soon as our bodies sense something, let's say food or disease, wheter by sight or smell, we begin to produce the enzymes necessary to digest & dispoae of it. This was shone to us, in 1980, in an updated experiment of Pavlov's dog (not the original canine)...You remember; bring food, ring a bell as the dog salivates, ring the bell and don't bring food and the dog still salivates. This is also the case with diseases, as soon as our bodies identifies a disease, it produces the defense neccessary to combat it, sight un-seen !!!

Well, in 1980, they also checked the composition of the saliva and SURPRISE, SURPRISE, SURPRISE, the enzymes in the saliva changed with the different meals. Current day studies are showing that our sense of smell is linked to weight

gain. If we smell a pastry, our system goes into storage mode...
(I gues I wasn't kidding when I joke at the local bakery - That
I am Here To Inhale All the Calories...)

So it is with Cancer, a cheeky little virus. In 1906, Doctor
John Stewart, of Scotland, showed us that our body's pancreas, produce - Proteolytic Enzymes (Protese, is the amino
acid involved), which distroy invading amino acids, whiich
viruses (like cancer) are made up of. He found this out by
grinding up the pancreas of farm animals, freshly killed on
the farm (people lived that way back then), and adminis-
tering it to terminally ill cancer patients, he cared for...Dr.
Stewart, was given a Noble Prize for his work and told to SKI-
DADDLE !!!

So WHY is Cancer so prevalent in our day & age ??? Nutrition, provided by diet, is the ammunition fortifying the
body's troops; for example a gun with ammunition is way more
letal, than without ammunition (and that's a fact-Jack) !!! The
GREATEST factor that weakens one's body's response is a poor
diet, devoid of proper nutrition.

In fact Cancer is so sneeky, that once avoiding the body's
defenses it settles into a cozy location to avoid further detec-
tion; behind the GUNK that poor nutrition does put into
the body....In the early 1930's, this Theory of Thromboplasts;
host cells and locations that Cancer settles into; getting cozy,
it sets up shop by forming a shell, so the body's defenses can
not penetrate and the rest becomes academic. If yous haven't
guessed, Yes, it was the same Dr. John Stewart, who received
another Noble Prize and was rode outta town on a rail...How
dare he cut into the medical professions profits, (which at
present date is 3 Trillion Dollars yearly just for Cancer Care)
by getting people healthy...

In speaking with a current (this year) medical school graduate, I was not surprised, but a bit flabbergasted (there's a word, I'll bet yous haven't heard in awhile); that in all the years of schooling in the medical discipline, there was still only three (3) WEEKS of instructions on Nutrition...In Business the saying is Location. Loction, Location; in Physiology - it is Nutrition, Nutrition, Nutrition, which is all of it according to our medical school graduate (well, at least 99.99% of it)...In this chapter I am going to bring to your attention to the raw power of Nutrition, so much so that the hairs on the back of your neck should be standing on end !!!

Okay, if yous have read my first book - Cooking for Mom and Pops -in it I state, that by changing my Mom's diet, I was able to ease certain problems, like colitis, which she suffered from for over 30 years. I was not able to find a Naturopathic doctor, so as to get a proper Bio-Nutrional Analysis for her, making me work in the blind with her.

After my Mom pasted into the next life, I was able to find a doctor, for my Pops, so as to get a partial - 80% - Bio-Nutritional Analysis from a urine test. With this I was able to set his nutrional intake, with supplements and diet. Within a few weeks, he was seeing better, even though he had macular degeneration for a few years; he was able to hear better, where, before you could be talking right to him, with no response; his walking improved, where as the day we first went to see this doctor, a breeze almost knocked him over. The color in his skin came back, where as before he was as white as a sheet. His appetite was better; his grip was stronger, he wasn't as sleepy; there were so many all over improvements, that I can say - I got my Pops back !!!

Here's a few more stories; Eight years ago I was working as a cook for a retirement home of forty (40) nuns, where half of the residents resided in the infirmary. Through a chain of events, I ran the kitchen for a month, the month of February, were we had two (2) blizzards. I began changing around the menu to reflect, what I thought, a more nutritous diet and by the end of this month, the nuns were walking straighter, instead of swaying; there was a clarity in their eyes and color (reddish cheeks) returned to their faces. When I went upstairs to the infirmary, because I had forgotten something on their cart, I was able to lead the invalid nuns in song (and if I had another month, I'd probably have them up dancing the jig, most being from Ireland)...

While on one of my errands to the infirmary, I noticed one nun; whom years earlier was the head cook, when there were one hundred (100) nuns in residence. She was a cook's-cook, this nun would rise at 2 am to go into NYC's fish market, to select the fish for the day or to the butcher for the meat and the fruit & vegetable market, She did this seven (7) days a week for all the years she ran the kitchen, She and her staff of nuns and lay workers, would make all the baked goods from scratch, as if it were a hundred years ago, cooking for a family.

Now the first time I met this specific nun, it was 4 or 5 months earlier; I had arrived early and was having a cup of coffee, while facing the entry, which was right next to the elevator and whom do you think was being brought in on a gurny from a rehab-center ??? That's right, this little nun, I don't even think she weighed a hundred pounds.

Now, yous have to picture this in your head. I siping on a hot cup of coffee, she's on this gurny, about 15 feet in front of me, waiting for the elevator and breathing through an oxygen mask. She picks up her weak hand and starts to point at me. I pick up my finger and start pointing to myself, saying -"ME". She starts nodding her head and waving me over with that weak finger, As I approach her, I say -"Yes, sister can I help you ???

With her other hand, she lifts the oxygen mask and says to me (now, yous have to think this with a little Irish accent, being that a good number of nuns in residence, were from Ireland); "Yorre Mikel, arrent you ???" "Yes, sister, Have I done something ???"; was my response. "No, No, Mikel" she says to me, "Yorre Touch is known !!!" This has been the best compliment, I have had in my whole life, especially, after I found out who she was...

Now, to get back to the original thought; as I am walking down the hallway of the infirmary, towards the dinning room, I pass this nun's room and happen to look in. There is this little nun, standing up on her own, using her walker to walk out of her room, to the dinning room. I stop and say to her,"sister, you sholdn't be up on your own"...Her response to me was, "Mikel, I feel like walking on my own to the dinning room and by God, that's what I'm to do" !!! True Story...

I have already mentioned this, but deserves repeating...Six years ago, while at the Vet for a routine visit for my dogs; a Beagle and a Malamute Husky, the vet informs me that my husky has AIDS (Auto-Immune Deficency Syndrome). I said, "WHAT". So, when I get home, I start doing some research. I change their diet; eliminating all processed foods, dog biscuits, dry and can foods and start feeding them some mixed vegetables and cook real animal protein for them. I purchase a de-hydrator and make various jerky treats (no spices), for them. The next year when we return for their check-up - NO AIDS !

Four years ago, through a series of mis-fortunes, someone I was close to, was diagnosed with stage four lung cancer, while on the operating table (which means, his regular physican did not have a clue and upon finding out, suggested this person be DNR- do not resuscitate; (hence, his culpability). They start chemo and radiation treatments and this person is wiped out, barely gets his sea legs back when it's time for another treatment. This goes on week, after week and he had to begin breathing with an oxygen tank in tow.

Having some empathy for this family's suffering; I decide to do a little research and loe & behold, I find out that - Beets - you know those red ground vegetables that stain your hands and everything else; are very powerful when it comes to dealing with lung cancer....Ya see, miracles abound around us, not like in the movies with a Grand Fanfare, but in the smallest gesture; like Elijah, "feeling God's pressence in a still small whisper." (1 Kings19:12)

So, I pick up a handfull of beets, organic, of course, boil them, drain the water, mash them up with some garlic, mixed Italian seasoning and olive oil and bring it to this family with the instructions: just a tea spoon each day, preferrably on some lettuce or if necessary a cracker (stay away from simple starches, like crakers or pasta, because they feed viruses like Cancer). Apparently - BEETS - work so well in breaking up Cancer of the Lungs that it can clog up the liver in the process of elimination. By the end of this month, this person is recovering from his chemo and radiation treatments, in a day, if not two; singing, whistling, doesn't even need the oxygen tank (it actually is a bother) and Stupid, feels so good and starts eating pasta, again (three, four times a-day)...Well, they run out of - BEETS - the pasta continues to flow and the Cancer finishes the job...Case Closed !!!

Have yous ever seen that commercial ??? You know the one where the people eat something and their head - EXPLODES- Poof !!! Well get yourselves ready, because I am about to do that to yous here. I am guilty of building to a crescendo (isn't that a nice word), and gently getting yous to this point; it's no holds barred now...

Have yous ever heard of the - GENOME project ??? Yous have probably seen the commercials offering to find an individual's ancestry by using their DNA. This offer traces to the Genome project, where modern day geniologists have been able to trace the migratory pattern of humanity by using the DNA of archeological finds scattered around our earth.

Well, just recently, a native North American Indian tribe won a legal dispute with the United States Government, over the burial grounds and burial rite of the skeletal remains of an unknown person. The U.S. Governments arguement was that they should be denied because the skeletal remains, especially the skull did not resemble that of the ancestors of this native North American tribe.

Even though the skull was of an elongated shape, the native North American tribe argued that this must be one of their ancetors, even though their ancestors have been shone to have rounded skulls, because the remains were deiscovered in an area that this tribe was known to frequent. Well, the Native American tribe was found to be correct. How can this be; you ask yourselves, astonished !!!

It seems that three (3) to five (5) hundred thounsand years ago when this tribes (very long lost) ancestors crosed over into North America, that at a certain point, the tribe split. Some of this tribe went into the interior of North America, feeding mostly on animals, such as the buffalo; and some hugged along the coast, all the way down to the tip of South America, feeding mostly on seafood, such as claims, prawns and the like (starting the first SEE-FOOD buffet); and the rest became the first entrepenuers of the continent, starting the first Casino (even though this is an Italian word), but did not do well because as of yet there were no others to patronize them. Learning the valuable lesson in business: do not get ahead of demand...

Now: One (1) million years before this (give or take a day), there seems to have been a massive migration of people, now known as Homo-Sapiens (which losely translates to: one who has come to know himself) out of south central Africa, that traveled along the Atlantic coast, up and around, the Mediterranen Sea going down into India and up and around into Europe.

This group that makes its way into Europe, meets up with a group, that migrated a million years before them; from the same part of Africa...We have come to call these people - Neanderthals (I'll bet they had a lot of gruntting to catch up on)...The cooking of raw foods, is accredited as having a great impact in the aesthetic nature of our appearance, today...

Even though these two groups had some similarities, the differances where striking; caused by a million years of diverse evolution which was sustained by diverse food sources. The Neanderthals had stuck themselves up in the European continent, which was quite frozen at that time of the Earth's history. Their main source of foods were other animals and even themselves, in times of famine, waiting for the summer for

Fruits and Vegetables. (This was in the days before humanity understood Seed-time and Harvest). The, New & Improved, Homo-Sapiens, fresh out of Africa, whom had a bounty of food choices to nurish themselves on, eventually overtook the Neanderthal and this is why I can type on a computer, that you can be reading this Thesis...

Most of this information, came to me -"Via PBS" and is why I am dedicating ten (10%) percent of my revenues to local PBS stations which I feel privileged to view (and who are in need of it, because our current POTUS, who really should be an avid viewer, so as to be informed, has canceled their stipend). While watching the local PBS station, i happened upon a program showing animals, specifically chimpanzees (whom we share 99% of our DNA with) in the wild, going about their normal routine. You know, if you've seen this type of programs, showing chimpanzees picking their ears, rubbing their butts on the ground, using a branch to sctrach their backs (sounds familiar), eating bananas, chewing on leaves (not smoking them, yet)... All of a sudden this group of chimpanzees decides to add meat to their menu-du-jour and take off after this little Rhesus Monkey. They corner this poor little guy and tear him apart and eat him (must of been the appetizer).

I am starring at this scene and my "Little Grey Cells" begin to perculate. We normally think of Chimpanzees, with whom we share 99% of our DNA with, eating fruits and vegetations, I don't know about yous, but I have never thought of chimpanzees driving up to the local burger hut. We now know, that in times of famine, humans would cannabalize the youngest amongst themselves.

Here Is the Epiphany - What if there was an extended period of drought in that part of Africa, a few (3 to 5) million years from whence the early humans, called hominins, originated from and the primates, especially the chimpanzees, had no fruit and vegetation to eat, turning to other animals, like Rhesus Monkeys (or even their own), as a main food source. We have just seen how a million years seperated the Neanderthals and the Homo-Sapiens and how a few hundred thoussnad years seperated the native North American tribes, that the divergent food source cause such distinct differences.

What if this extented period of drought and change in food source created the missing link between Humans and Primates ??? SHAZBOT !!! My brain started shaking...(How's bout yours?) We now accredit cooking foods over a heat source as drastically changing the appearance of the species between the Hominid to Neanderthal Man to Homo-Sapiens to Whatever We Are Today (Homo-Novus ???)...I wasn't there, but this is very plausible...In "The Origen of the Species", Darwin noticed that a bird, that was denied a food source, by the other birds - changed the shape of it's beak to enable it to go after another food source...

The Body is Truely Capable of Incredible Things, if the Mind will let it; we see this in evolution... The Power of Nutrition !!!

CHAPTER 7

SEVEN (7) : A TRUELY DIVINE NUMBER

SEVEN (7); THE winner, craps the looser...Three sevens (777) Jackpot...On the Seventh Day God rested from his labors (da-ya think he cracked open a cold one, maybe knosched a lit-tle)???. If I haven't all ready taxed your minds so your brains are throbbing, then this chapter should do it. There are Seven Continents...There are Seven Seas...There are Seven (7) Chakras...There are Seven (7) Systems that comprise the Human body...And there are Seven (7) Dwarfs (can you name them???)

In this very chapter, we are getting into (1) the Seven - 7 - Days to fat burning, (2) the human circadian rythm of Seven - 7 - Years and (3) the Seventh -7th - Sense....(what should be playing in your heads right now is the musical theme, played on the theramin, from the original Star Trek)..,

The first seven, to speak of, is the - Seven Days to Fat Burning. It takes the human body Seven (7) Days to get to Fat Burning; ; I keep on repeating this point so's it will sink in. This is IT !!! This is how we are wired. This is why 98 % of diets FAIL. This is why most all diets are slow in weight lose. This is why when we fall off a diet, the body easily gains weight again.

When I was in the second (2nd) grade, I weighed 172 lbs., and I have never been under that weight since. School, ruined my figure; until kindegarten I was a normal child and I have the pictures to prove it. Then I started school (which I had to be dragged into by my Pops and his two younger brothers) and discovered soda and chips and the worst, being sedentary. Until then, I ran about ALL-DAY; in the course of a day I had to sit still and listen for most of the day, then sit most of the night to do home-work. I went to a Holy Rosary Catholic grammer school and there was a ton of home-work (this is why I was a power-lifter, later in life).

Like most young boys, when I started noticing girls I thought it a good idea to slim down abit. I would spend the whole week watching what I ate, losing 2; 3; maybe 4 pounds; then the weekend would come and on Saturdays i would walk down the long block (apparently-not long enough) to Central Bakery for the dinner-bread and of course, my favorite Pizza-Foccacia; which is simply a round pan bread baked with plum tomatos squezzed into it. I love this so much, that when we moved from Union City, so did Central Bakery, to the town right next to us... (Temptation seems to follow me)...

On Sundays, it would be pan-cakes for breakfast; Pasta, with meat sauce and Bread for lunch; and a free-for-all in the fridge for supper (so much for losing weight). This would go on every week; what fustration. Instead of getting good attendance medals, I should of been given the Edison-medal; for doing the same thing over & over without success.

So, Why did this not work ??? Because - It Is SEVEN Days to FAT-burning !!! The moment we put a simple starch (like grains) in our mouths, (even the sense of smell); our body SHUTS down FAT BURNING and goes to Fat-STORAGE.. That is correct; it is our body's defense mechanism to combat starvation. When we do not place a simple starch (like grains) in our mouths, our body begins the process of Self-Preservatiom and begins to let lose some stored water, for the first (3) three days. the next (3) three days the body gives up some muscle; then on the Seventh (7th) Day, God rested from his labors (Genesis 2:2); but our body gets a move on and begins to burn fat.

Now, that's the fact - Jack; this is why 98 % of weight lose diets fail. soon as you put a simple starch in your mouth - Fat Burning, shuts OFF and Fat Storage turns ON. Hence, the constant se-saw of weight lose and the worst news is that Fat LOSE is proportional, while Fat GAIN is SPECIFIC... What ever weight we loose, we loose all over the body at the same time...Hence, when we loose weight, wheter it be 2 or 20 pounds; this lose is all over the body. When we gain weight, our body stores it is specific places; hence, giving our body a dis-pro-portionate look.

Becoming civilized has a great deal to do with this. Approximately fifteen thousand (15,000) years ago, humanity learned a great secret; the Bible calls it - "seedtime and harvest"(Genesis 8:22). Until then humanity was a hunter-gatherer; we ate what we caught or found. Humanity was mostly nomadic, traveling to different parts to find food. "I am telling you the truth; a grain of wheat remains no more than a single grain unless it is dropped into the ground and dies. If it does die, then it produces many grains."(John 12:24)... (Remember this verse because it will become a lynch-pin for the Atruistic Diet.)

We may also thank the Earl of Sandwich, circa mid-1700's, for inventing the first Grab-n-Go meal, by placing his food between two hunks of bread and distorting the ratio of bread to meat in a meal. Until then, most people ate larger quantities of meats and vegetables, using bread, as an accompanyment, to scoop up their meal or a sponge to sop up the juices,

Let us now speak of the next seven (7); the Seven (7) Year Circadin Rythm of the human body. In a Seven (7) Year Period, the human body re-places each and everyone of its cells. The re-placements are made up of whatever it is you are, or are not, putting into your body. The better your nutrition, the better building materials your body has to use. The better building materials - the better one's health...We, very much, are what we EAT...

What also affects our bodies is what we do not put into it !!! Surprising; Ahey ??? Our bodies need the many Vitamins and Minerals that are found, and are Bio-Available, in Fruits, Nuts, Vegetation, Legumes and Meats; which the lack of causes illnesses. Did you know that a lack of Magnesium can cause heart arythmia and that a lack of Lithium, a trace mineral found in Vegetation, is responsible for Bi-Polarism or Manic/Depressive (no not Demons)... I thought that was a mental disease ? Yes. a mental disorder brought on by a continual lack of nutrition...

In our day & age we now know that Bi-Polarism (or Manic/Depression) is caused by a lack of Lithium in the diet. Lithium is a trace mineral, found in Vegetation... We would have less Arrogance and Homelessness in the world and our leaders, if so many more people would just - EAT THEIR GREENS !!!

This begins in-utero, with the mother's nutrition. The better nutrition ingested, the better for the fetus. The lack of nutrition, becomes detremental to the fetus. (Ezekial 18:1 - "When the parents eat unripe grapes, the children's teeth suffer.) There are many modern day studies which correlate poor nutrition, with problems with the new-born and good nutrition, with healthy development of the new-born.

We are well aware that a lack of good nutrition is responsible for ADD (attention deficeit disorder), ADHD (attention deficeit hypertensive disorder) and JAJ (just a jerk, which many of us suffer from)...Modern day mothers are very aware of this and are making great stides to obtain optimal nutrition, for themselves, as well as for their children.

In the Bible, I have exculpated (there's a word worth a buck) a Jacob's Blessing, that relates to nutrition. Jacob was the second of twins, who usurps, his brother, Esau's blessing (as we have seen earlier) over a pottage of Lentils & some chicanery... Later in life (just before Jacob is to kick the bucket) in Genisis 48:14, Jacob purposelly switches his hands to give the blessing to Ephram, Joseph's younger son...

Well I have noticed this to be so, with the second child in the family...I believe, that till the first child is conceived, the woman, always watching her figure does without eating properly or even at all. Studies show that rats die when kept on the diet of an average female college student. So, the first child suffers a lack of development because of this...Where, with the second child, now the woman has been eating better and is enriched by the better nutritional intake...

One can take a group of outdoor animal and feed them a processed food diet and watch how every subsequent litter develops distortions and anomalies. I told this to a self considered; "smart" relation, whoses response was - well they all having sex with each other (FYI: that's what they do in the real world, too)...Taking the last liter and reversing the process, feeding them what they would normally feed on in the wild, by the tenth generation, they are back to normal (don't yous just Love this stuff ???)...

It goes without saying, that there is a MONUMENTAL effort to improve the quality of nutrition in schools all over the United States...We have finally come to the realization that the BETTER we feed the children, the BETTER their scholastic performance will be; hence less problems in adult life...The Food Network and PBS stations have been at the forefront of this, especially with adults, in aiding and guiding BETTER Food chioces !!!

Also, the purer the Mother's nutrition, the cleaner and crisper the senses of the newborn. It is well documented and I personally know of two children, whom upto 3 or 4 years, could see spirits in their house. People would say as they grow older - they grow out of it. Not so fast, Sherlocks; as they grow older they are ingesting foods that calcify or occlude (cover over) the pineal gland (aka; the third eye)...Yep, the same little gland (the size of a pea) that is responsible for the release of melatonin, that allows us to drift of to slumber-land, is respomsible for aiding us in peering beyond the vail (but more about this later)... FLURIDE (also occuldes) - which is in tooth paste and our water...Co-in-si-dence ??? NOT !!! The Dark side controling the situation...

Until the 20th century, the daily challange was just getting food and the food was seasonal, which means a whole lot of the same product at the same time and filler(BREADS) for the rest of the time. The world was basicsally an agrarian culture, revolving around harvests. A plethora of fruits and vegetables in late summer and early autumn, but not so much the rest of the year. Preserving of these aided in providing them during the year, but they weren't fresh.

The Great Challenge of our day is - CHEMICALS (BEES) & GENETIC MODIFICATION !!!

Chemicals cause distortions in our genetic code (or make-up), also, killing off 50 % of the Bee population and Genetic Modification provides an un-complete product (kind of like getting a car missing 3 tires, or no engine or the seats are missing or the hood, trunk and steering wheel is missing). I believe you have the picture. Two paragraphs ago, the studies I mentioned were on animals. The Human studies you are seeing unfold before your eyes, in current time. Along with being the wealthiest country ever in the history of this earth; we have inherited the diseases of the wealthly and have the sickest society ever.

"I keep my promise for thousands of generations and forgive evil and sin; but I will not fail to punish children and grandchildren to the third ond fourth generatuon for the sins of their parents."(Exodus 34:7)...This is Very True of Nutrition...May God continue to Bless those Good Souls who provide care and funds for the infirm and needy...

What about that Seventh (7) Sense, I've mentioned...What do you think it is ??? We all Know the Five (5) Senses, (right ???); Hearing, Smell, Sight, Taste, Touch (kinda like naming the seven dwarfs or Santa's eight reindeer)...The senses of smell, sight, and taste, definately are involved in our digestive process; if yous re-collect the updated Pavlov Dog experiment I've mentioned. Hearing and touch may have some periphery effect on digestion.

Do you have a Sixth (6) Sense; an intuition, a power of perception apart from the other Five (5) Senses. The kind of intuition or psychic ability that would allow a certain lovely young woman to ask a patron, who comes for coffee, once, sometimes, twice a week, if all is well ??? Remembering that encounter, over a month later, without being prompted, because it was on the customer's mind (Interesting)...Telling that customer that she'd be transferring to another store; a store that was already on this customer's mind to start patronizing - Very Interesting, Indeed !!! The kicker is; she is Vegan & somewhat psychic...

It is apparent that women have a greater ability for intuition & being psychic, and I believe, that this is because women are usually watching their weight & figure and tend to include into their diets a greater amount of Fruits & Vegetables (and less of the white stuff; sugar, salts, starches) keeping the synapses clearer, tending them to be more intuitive...

Although, I can never guess what's on a woman'a mind; It seems that women can always guess what's on my mind !!! Ah Women; there was a great stroke of creation for you, probably the best the Big-Guy has done; although not perfect, but nothing He's done has been so, yet...

Actually, I am a bit Psychic (although, I'll tell people that I am psychodic, for a chuckel)... Many a times, I'll be thinking of something or watching TV and a thought of a program or song, I haven't heard nor seen in a while comes to mind and within a few days, I'll hear that song on the radio or see that TV program. This is all independent of any advertizing or program listing.

A little more, out in left field; I'll be watchung TV and an actor comes to mind, again, independent of what I am or have wacthed recently, with the thought - I haven't seen nor heard of so-n-so in a while, I wonder what they've been up to !!! Within a few days or a week, that person is announced as having died...This has happened with John Gandolfini, Yvonne

Craig (the original Bat-Girl), John Semore Hoffman, Carrie Fischer and Debbie Reynolds (a double-header), Jerry Lewis (just recently), to name just a few. People Who were not sick, nor in the news for anything and POOFF, gone. (This almost happened with Harison Ford, but he survived his plane crashing, although, he keeps on trying).

What about over the fence and into the meadows ??? Have you ever dreamed of some thing and months later have it come to fruitition ??? Months before, each one of my dogs pasased away, I would have a similar dream; of them running away from me (this just happened with Chelsea a few months ago) and no matter how hard I try, I can't regain them... Crystal, Luiza, Chelsea, were not ill or sick or injured at the time of those dreams...There is some thing to be said about a pre-appointed time to leave; maybe it is, so as to return at a pre-appointed time; at least that is how I console myself...

Dogs also have an intuition (almost, that they can read our minds), in that, I noticed that their behavior changed. They usually go about doing what all dogs normally do; but weeks before passing on, they would stop, look up and take in the scenary, the view, as if to cherish it for a last time...

Have Yous ever spoken Faith over someones life, without realizing It ??? This has happened to me with a few people, such as close friends...One instance, almost forty (40) years ago, I was with a friend (brother), I graduated high school with. I had just introduced this person to a local fraternal organization (who is still a vibrant member, to this day) and we were discussing our differing successes in dating. I didn't even realize what was coming out of my mouth. (I Says) - I'll bet, that one of these cronies takes a likin to you and brings you home to meet his daugther, were yous fall for each other, gets married and haves a reall good life together..." Sure as the Pope is Catholic, that's just what happend...

Another instance is with another high school friend (brother); when the woman he Loves, leaves him for another, my mouth just said-"if she is the person you think she is, then she will be drawn back to your Love. Just continue being a friend to her (being that they worked together)... In all justice, I can not take all the credit for this Epiphany; a gallon of red table wine happened to be the catalysist...God is Good !!!

I began becoming aware of this on September 10, 2001, which started out as any other day. I was retired at the time, between buisnesses, as one would say and I awoke, I had breakfast, went about my daily routine, but as I did so I became increasingly agigated, to the point, by that evening I could not sit still. Something, I did not know what, was eating me up from within. It was a Monday evening and I decided to go into NYC, which I rarely did on a Monday, unless one of my visiting-friends had come to town. I visited my usual places and on the way home I stopped for a red light on 72nd & Broadway, in front of the Grey Papaya (I always catch that light, for some reason) and The City was deserted. Literally, there was no one around and I just got this eerie-feeling, like something was up or going to happen.

The next morning I was awoken to the sound of loud radios of people sitting in lawn chairs, across from my house watching the World Trade Center Atrocity. I lowered my American-flag to half mast, went to the local church, said some prayers and lit a few candles, tried to donate blood, but was turned away, due to the blood station being overwhelmed and then understood...

Another instance was, a few years ago, I went to the movies and arrived early as is my custom...The previews had not yet started and so I was noticing the people that were entering and taking their seats. A thought came to me - "that it wouldn't take much for someone to come in and shot up the place"... Wouldn't you know; later that evening, in Colorado, a gunman did just that at the Batman premiere...

As I am preparing this book for publishing, going over things; a thought crossed my mind - "that with all the terrorist stuff going on, why no one had tried anything in Las Vegas"... Three days later - it happened...Doesn't send a chill up your spine ???

How important is nutrition in developing this sense ??? "Prove thy servants, I beseech thee, ten (10) days and let them give us pulse to eat and water to drink...And at the end of the ten (10) days their countenance appeared fairer and fatter in flesh, than all the children which ate the portion of the king's meat...As for these four children, God gave them knowledge and skill in all learning and wisdom; and Daniel had understanding in all visions and dreams," (Daniel 1 12, 15 & 17)

The Seventh (7) Sense; the ability to peer behind and beyond the vail of unknown. "and it shall come to pass afterward, that I will pour out my spirit upon all flesh and your sons and your daughters shall prophecy, your old men shall dream dreams, and your young men shall see visions". (Joel 2:28)

What part does Nutrition have in opening this seventh (7) Sense ??? Do yous remember, that I have previously mentioned how someone inadvertantly mentioned, eating a bowl of Lentils, often as a child, and now, as an adult, is using the Seventh (7) Sense in healing ???

It's all about nutrition !!! There is no mistaking how those who fast and abstain from food; have these cathartic events. The Buddha, sits under a sacred tree, fasting and comes up with the tenets of Buddhism... Along with Martin Luther & Saint Francis, also, avid actectics (whether by choice or force) and even Muhammid, in the cave, probably went without food...

"Then Jesus, was led by the Spirit into the desert to be tempted by the devil (the Arch-Angel Samel or Satan-in the Greek or Lucifer-in the Latin, light bearer), he fasted for forty (40) days and nights and afterwards he was hungry. The tempter approached and said to him, if you are the Son of God. command that these stones become loaves of bread..."(Mathew 4:1-3) And Jesus answered: What, No smear...

Look, the very first temptation - BREAD...When I was a youth My Mom & Me would have a piece of day old Italian Loaf Bread, dipping it into a hot cup of coffee, my mouth drools just thinking of it. Did Jesus know that BREAD was also a sensory blocker. Yesterday I had Pancakes for breakfast, Italian hero for lunch and this morning I am all foggy-headed. As an experiment, for two (2) weeks I ate starches at every meal, which resulted in me coming down with a cold, in a time of year when colds are not prevalent.

I do not recommend fasting !!! The first thing that happens when one fasts is that the brain goes into - hypoglycemic shock; the brain becomes starved of the sugar, it so desperately uses for fuel. This is why all addictions are sugar based. Depriving the brain of fuel begins the spasming of the electrical circuitry in our heads and all kinda things begin to happen, the most common, of which is hallucinations. How many times have you heard others speak of cathartic events while fasting; this is a big-hit on the bible stumping circuit during revivals making the outcomes subject to skepticism.

Also, I do not recommend fasting because so many people do not understand the health inplications. It is important to understand how to prepare to enter a fast and even more important on how to come out of a fast; some have died because they over-did it...I have already mentioned fasters, such as Buddha; Jesus; Gandi was a well known faster and Pythagoras formed a society of mathematicians who regularly fasted and I'll bet you did not know that Andrew Jackson, the seventh President of the United States, fasted for medical reason of severe pain caused by a bullet he received during a duel and that Hippocrates, the Father of Modern Medicine, said - "let Food be your medicine & your medicine be your Food", also prescribed fasting as a means to cleanse the body of impurities...

Why Fast ??? One can gently cleanse the body of its impurities by adhering to this Altruistic Diet !!! It does not make sense to me, to go through the sufferings & pains of fasting, just to return to a diet that made one need to fast from it, in the first place...

Through out history fasting has been used to offset the excesses of a bountyfull lifestyle (along with leaches, take your choice)...Muhammid was known to have a festering sore, upon his back; which back then was interpeted as a sign of a being a prophet (probably made up after the fact)...

I had a cyst on my back (turned out to be an ingrown hair, which my wonderful cousin, Maria, popped (who also happens to be intuitve, calling me, just after I proof read this part, wondering if I should include her name...Thank You !!!);

does that make me a see-er, at least ??? Muhammid was also known to have Severe Halitosis (Bad Breath), that he would have honey before being with one of his thirteen wives. Life is Good !!! Also, all signs of an extravagant lifestyle, lots of Meats and no Vegetables...

Some societies, Like the ancient Romans, would have vomitoriums; but the acids for the stomach would wear away the enamel of the teeth and cause severe bad breath. This also happened to my cousin, who happened to eat himself to death, with no assistance from his family, who tried all these fads to no avail. I shared my diet with him; he smiled, threw it away and died nearly two years later.

If yous think about it, every day we go into and come out of a fast; hence this is why our first meal in the morning is called - Break-Fast...Then, if any of yous are like myself, that when I arise during the night, I will usually have some fruit and nuts, (or that left over pizza, that just won't see the light of day). I have found that fresh fruit during the evening and/ or over night - Super Charges, my dreams (especially plums) The correct fuel, for the brain, gives it the energy needed, while at rest, to begin peering behind the vail; begging the question - What else is there ???

Have you ever been led by the Holy Spirit ??? Let me share with you...A few years ago, at Christmas time, I was shopping at the local discount retailer (Daddy War-Bucks, I am not) and happened upon a cut-out sign that reads:"God is Good". I purchased it and hung it over my rear doorway, so's once in awhile, it would remind me that God is Good; it's a simple enough thought. A few months later, while walking my dogs, I began thinking that if one would add an - o - to God it would read Good and if one took away an - o - from Good it would read God. Interesting, AHEY, (all the world's problems should be this simple)...Now, three or four months after this I happened to order -"the Gospel of Mary Magdalen", and while reading this it became apparent that in it, Jesus continually refers to God, as The Good.

Here's another for yous; on November 12, 2014, I decided to register with the Universal church as a Non-Denominational Minister. Two (2) days later, while sitting on the toilet (this is where all the great stinker, I mean thinkers, pondered) a tile on my bathroom wall began to become aparent to me. Let me prefice this by saying that these tiles have been on this bathroom wall since 1979 (yep, 35 years). A liitle round nose became apparent and above it eye sockets and a brow above that, beneath was a beard with a mouth and from the mouth a breath, forming four quadrants, like a heart, and a cross in the middle. Above the head seems to be a bird in flight, with a flame extending from one wing tip to the other wing tip. For thirty five (35) years I have been starring (sometimes concentrating) at the Trinity... (SHAZ-BOTT)...Just that this tile exists, blows me away, and that it wound up on my bathroom wall and right in front of me, so's I can reach out and touch it; leaves me shaking my head, (to listen to the rattling)...This tile could have been placed upside down or anywhere else on the wall and I most probably would never have noticed it.

I have also come to realize that this same - Holy Spirit - is not only my mentor, but my protector. Back in fifth (5) grade, I remember playing kick ball, at grammer school. I was running towards first base and just happened to stop, in my tracks, before I reached it. Coming at me, at all out speed, was this kid in my class. He ran right past me, hit the ten foot beveled metal fence (I don't know how many of yous remember these), full-blast...The fence, ricocheted him onto his back and he had knocked himself out...Will Wonders Never Cease !!! As I look back over my life, I can remember many more stories such as this...

I have been told, that my accomplishments and failures are all meant to lead me to fullfill my assignment or purpose on this earth and in this lifetime. I have come to realize this, in looking back over my life; hence, my dedication, at the beginning of this work (if yous haven't read it, yous may wish to look it over)...Even with my girlfriends, I realized it is probably meant that I do not marry in this lifetime, so I can finish this second book, in my trilogy (the next book will be even more interesting)...In looking back, it is way to coincedental, that every time I would begin to think of getting more serious or proposing marriage, events would take place that seperated us. My last girlfriend, got a promotion and salary doubling and moved half way across the U.S.,within two weeks... Oh Well, saved again !!!

This Altruistic Diet, gently clenses the body (clensing receptors & transmitters) and in doing so, Awakens the Senses; eventually the Seventh Sense. I have previously mentioned that - Benjamin Franklin was a Vegetarian (because of frugality) and look what he accomplished, just think how much further he could of gone, if he did not eat Bread (Bread. that very thing we are told to eat, back in Genesis 3:19, as a punishment)...If we could clear our systems of the GUNK, then maybe, we too can talk to and understand the animals, like Dr, Doolittle...

What do you think is behind those who can see spirits or angels about us ???

What energy do you think is behind the Quija board and the movement that goes about, without touching it ???

What do you think it means to see someone's aura or the vibrations, of the rainbow (the ever-present Energy, in our atmosphere, about us; which is actually a Circle, a SPHERE) without it having rained ??? That same Energy that the Arch of the Covenant, an excellant electrical conductor, being a wooden box, inlaid and encased in Gold, absorbed...

Pythagoras did extensive research into the vibrations in musical notes and how they correspond in physics. Vibrations which make up the sounds, which come from our vocal cords. Vibrations which make up everything in existence. Vibrations that get damped down with a heavy diet, one that clogs-up our system(s). Vibrations that Vibrate with Vitality, with an ALTRUISTIC DIET...

Benjamin Franklin knew of this energy and demonstrated it with his famous kite in a lightning storm, that electrified a key, that key that illuminates our imagination, that very thing that seperates us from our chimpanzee cousins at the 17th chain of our DNA... That Energy, that has been tugging at the coat-tails of humanity, eversince; before there was - The Word, there was thought of the Word and thoughts are energy that move faster than the speed of light.. $E = M \times C2$...

Things that make one go, HHHMMMMM !!! "There is more under heaven and upon earth, than can be imagined in your simple philosophy, my dear Horatio..." (Shakepeare's-Hamlet)

C H A P T E R   8

THE GREAT INSPECTOR CLUES-OH !!!

WE ARE ABOUT to use -"Our Little Grey Cells"- which is actually a favorite phrase of my favorite literary inspector; the unimitatable Belgian Inspector Hercule Poriot...We are going to go back to Chapter 2 and place all of the clues under a magnifying glass; like Sherlock Holmes. Seeing them for what they are, using the knowledge we have gained, we will eliminate the improbale, leaving us, the truth...

Fasten your seatbelts cause this is the quick-money, triple bonus point round, where I will set up a chart of buzz-words from the out takes back in chapter 2 (feel free to go back and consult),,,We are first going to answer the Question - WHERE...

Exodus 2:5

KJV - Moses fled to Midian...GN - Moses fled to Midian...ASB - Moses fled to Midian...ACB - Moses fled to Midian...

Exodus 3:11

KJV - Moses leeds Jethro's flock to the mountain of God - Horeb...GN - one day leeds Jethro's flock to Mt. Sinai...ASB - to Horeb, mountain of God leeds Jethro's flock...ACB - leeds Jethro's flock to Horeb, mountain of God...

Exodus 15:2

KJV - Elim, 12 wells & 70 palm trees...GN - come to Elim, 12 wells & 70 palm trees...ASB - come to Elim, 12 wells & 70 palm trees...ACB - Elim, 12 wells & 70 palm trees...

Exodus 18:5

KJV - Jethro came to Moses encampment at the mount of God...GN - Jethro came to Moses at the Holy Mount...ASB - Jethro came to Moses' encampment at the mountain of God... ACB - Jethro came to Moses's encampment at the mountain of God...

Exodus 19:2

KLV - they departed Rephidim...GB - they left Rephidim... ASB - they set out from Rephidim... ACB - journeyed from Rephidim...

Galatians 4:25

KJV - Agar, Mt.Sinai in Arabia...GN - Hagar stands for Mt. Sinai in Arabia...ASB - now Hagar is Mt.Sinai in Arabia...ACB - Hagar, Mt.Sinai in Arabia...

Do you understand this last piece from Galatians, written (supposedly) by St. Paul -aka (also known as) -Saul from Tarus, Italy - a big deal Rabbi who wanted to muscle in on the Jerusalem turf...When I shared this information to an Egyptian-Coptic Christian, who is 15 years older (not wiser) than me; his eyes bugged out, his ears turned red and kept on insisting that Sinai was in Egypt and then made the mistake of asking me - How do you explain this???

I just looked at him and said - "They Lied !!!" Ya see, I lost two (2) years searching in the wrong place (kinda like Indiana Jones, who knowning the correct information, found the tomb). Once I stumbled upon the correct location of the Hebrews, it all came together.

In Exodus 2 - Moses goes to Midian, which is modern day Saudi Arabia. In Exodus 3 - Moses takes a stroll with a flock (be careful whom you associate with) of sheep/goats. In my bible, I have a map and that map shows that from the tip of the Gulf of Aqaba (which seperates Egypt and Saudi Arabia) to where Mt. Sinai is in Egypt, it is approximately 200 mile walk (give or take); south west; which is quite an accomplishment with a flock of sheep in tow, no water, no grass, all that baaaing. YECK !!!

It just so happens (and this is what i stumbled upon, in the two (2) years I wandered) that Jethro, Moses' father-in-law, is from a smal town named Al Bad, in Saudi Arabia (Midian) , where he is still venerated to this day. This Al Bad, happens to be 10 to 15 miles from a mountain called Jebelel Lawz, which by chance has a reddish top...Do yous think that, maybe, the burning bush was mistaken for the reddish mountain top and maybe Ezra and his Written-Rabis got it wrong or embelished (I like that word)...Now Al Bad is approxinately two (2) hundred miles, south east, from the tip of the Lake of Aqaba; so we're talking approximately a 400 mile walk, with a flock of sheep (that's quite a stretch of the leg and imagination), if Moses made the trip to Sinai, in Egypt form Al Bad...

In Exodus 20, Moses receives the Commandments on the Holy Mount. In Exodus 18, Jethro of Midian, comes to meet

Moses (and the rest of the shi-bang), which happened to be encamped at Rephidim, as we see in Exodus 19:2, being a few more miles to the east of Al Bad. In Exodus 15, we have the Hebrews in Elim (where there are psalm trees & wells of water, which means moisture) which is in Saudi Arabia on the way to Al Bad and Horeb, the mountain of God; also, the Manna manifestation occurs (which is Exodus 16)...I'd bet dollars for donuts that Mt.Sinai (Horeb or Hagar)) is really in Saudi Arabia and not Egypt - SURPRISE-SURPRISE-SURPRISE !!!

And now for the - WHY...

Genisis 1:29

KJV - Herbs bearing seed, trees yielding fruit with seed as meat...GN - all kinds of Grains, all kinds of fruit. for animals & birds grass & green leaf vegetables...ASB - every plant yielding seed & every tree with seeds in fruit as food...ACB - every seed bearing plant & every tree with fruit bearing seeds...

Genesis 9:3

KJV - every living thing, every green herb...GN - eat all animals & birds, as well as green plants... ASB - every moving thing for food and green plants...ACB - every moving creature, also green plants as food...

In the GN version of Gen 1:29; the word - GRAINS - was that word that set me adrift for two years. I happen to have and read the Good News version, since it was given to me on my SEARCH weekend forty (40) years ago. When I first looked up - grains in the bible - I received back - barley, corn, millet, rye, wheat. The only one indigenous to Egypt (where Mt.Sinai is suppose to be) is Millet. Simple; Right ??? Too simple, because when you study millet's effect on the human body, it makes us - Hypothyroidic (slows down the metabolism), it gives us goiter, making the body iodine deficent. Remember what I wrote way back, about - NOT BEING ABLE TO DIGEST GRAINS; it gums-up-da-body... Not Good...

Then, I happened upon the word - SEED - in one of the other versions - HAZZA, illumination. Well now we're talkin - you can have seeds from fruit, seeds from trees - NUTS (to you)... Wether to sprout your NUTS by soaking them, to activate the DNA or nutrition, is still being debated. If yous soak your - NUTS - they may get soft & muschy...So try not to soak your - NUTS -to long.

Next we get to the - WHAT...("he's on second...I'm not asking you who's on second...who's on first...I don't know...oh, he's on third") - Sorry, I just couldn't pass it up...

Exodus 16:31

KJV - Manna, looks like corriander seed, white;tastes like wafer with honey...GN - Manna, small white seed;tastes like cakes made with honey...ASB - Manna, like corriander seed, white; tastes like wafer made with honey...ACB - Manna, white corriander seed;tastes of honey...

Numbers 11:7

KJV - Manna, like corriander seed; color of bdellium...GN - Manna was like small seeds, whitish-yellow in color...ASB - Manna, like corriander seeds, appearance like bdellium... ACB - Manna, was like corriander seeds, appearance of bdellium...

Yous are probably wondering what the word - bdellium - is ???
The color of - bdellium - is amberish (or a reddish-orange or
a rust). Corriander seeds which are a browish-yellow...This is
to say an off brown, maybe a kaki; as opposed to a brownish-
yellow, which would be a not so bright yellow. Like a beige,
like corriander seeds. Either way, Manna, is NOT a frost
like flake - IT IS A SEED !!! LENTIL !!! Specifically - Yellow
Lentils, which, by the way, isn't really yellow, but beige and is
indigenous to Midian (where Moses and his circus really was),
or Saudi Arabia (for you contemporaries)...

And now for the - HOW (and How)...

Exodua 16: 13,14 & 15

KJV - dew lay about Manna...GN - dew fell upon camp, dew
evaporates...ASB - dew lay on ground, fine flakes like hoar-
frost...ACB - morning dew gone up, fine flake like thing...

Numbers 11:8

KJV - dew, Manna fell upon it...GN - Manna, fell with dew,,,ASB
- dew fell, Manna fell with it...ACB - dew and Manna fell with it...

Numbers 11:9

KJV - ground in mills, beat in mortars, baked in pans, made
cakes of it, taste of fresh oil... GN - grind it or pound it into
flour, boil it or make it into flat cakes, tasted like baked bread
with olive oil...ASB - ground it in mills, beat it in mortars,
boiled in pots, made cakes taste of olive oil...ACB - ground
between mill stones, beat in mortars, boiled in pots, made
into loaves, tasted like cakes made with olive oil...

Okay, we have two processes here; hence is why is Chapter (1) One, I mention baking and cold preperation of the Lentils. Now, if the Hebrews were in the desert, I sincerly doubt there may have been some morning dew, but (there is always a but), because they were near Elim which had 12 wells and 70 psalm trees. A little oasis, so to say and where there is water, there is moisture & there is dew. So, Moses was probably discribing the process of sprouting the Lentil Seeds; leaving then in water (or morning dew, not for too long because they'll get funky) so's they are easier to work with. Just in the way out possibility that there was morning dew, it is possible that the Hebrews laid thier seeds out over night to soak up what ever moisture was available; hence, the hoar-frost. This is what we see in Exodus 16: 13 & Number 11:8...

In Number 11:9, we see whole other process - grounding between mill stones, pounding in mortars, making it into flour; boiled in pots (da furst Bagels), tasted like cakes made with olive oil and (back up some to Exodus 16:31) wafers made with honey...The wife, of a friend of mine's from high school, every Christmas gives me peanut brittle. One Christmas I had this passage in mind and peanut brittle in hand and my little grey cells began to perculate. What's to say that the Hebrews, didn't mixed some honey with the sprouted Lentils, spread it out on their heated pans or stones, let it cool down and snapped them up into snacks (maybe the first trail-mix) !!!

Here's the WHEN...

Exodus 16:16

KJV; GN; ASB; ACB - gather an Omer for each person each day and twice that before the Sabbath...

Exodus 16:22

KJV - bake today, seethe what remaineth...GN - bake today...
ASB - bake and boil, what you will...ACB - bake and boil what
you will...

An Omer is equivalent to a Liter and to Seethe is to boil (that
should help yous some)...Now a liter of Lentil Seed is approximately the size of a loaf; so each person would have a loaf to
eat each day. I don't know about yous, but I do not eat a loaf of
bread per day. It takes me about a week to eat a loaf of bread;
so a loaf of Lentils, would be quite filling...

Now I am going to put it all together for YOUS for ease, to
see the flow... Okay !!!

- Moses leaves Egypt and makes his way to Midian (mod-
  ern day Saudi Arabia), marries Jethro's, the chief priest,
  daugther...
- 40 years later, Moses returns to Egypt and leads the
  Hebrews out of captivity...
- On the way, near Elim, God sends Manna (Lentils) and
  Quail (birds) for food.
- Jethro, Moses' father-in-law comes (from Al Bad) to
  Rephidim to meet up with the Hebrews.
- Moses recives the commandments at Hagar (or Horeb) -
  the mountain of God (Jebel El Lawz)...

This is the abbreviated version...Fairly simple, Ahey ???

The Webster's dictionary, defines - ALTRUISTIC - as : interests in accordance with ethical purposes; or the American Heritage dictionary (which I perfer) defines - ALTRUISTIC - concern for the welfare of others, Selfless...The later definition, keeping in the theme of a COMPASSIONATE Creator, a Father figure (if you will) whose Love is Selfless, doing things for his others... "...and there was not a man to till the ground" KJV-Genisis 2:5...It doesn't much sound like man was crerated out of Love (as the Religions fill our ears with), but out of a need to have a grounds keeper; and then he created Adam (remember, after the day of rest), the first Hebrew and his lineage, where supposed to be sod-busters. So the eating from the forbidden tree was a SET-UP, from the very start. Now we know WHY the tree was there, actually, and that the Arch-Angel Samel (aka., Satan; aka., Lucifer) was in KA-HOTS with the "God-Da-Father"; doing the bidding of the Capo-de-Tutti-Capi, makiing them two youngsters - "an offer, they don't refuse"...

Whatever the Truth really is (your guess, is as good as mine), we have a magnaminous gesture from nature to us, in the form of a proper nutrition for humanity. All, we really need is under our nose, we need only reach out (or roll a cart down the shopper's aisle) and have our way with it. In the final analysis, it really is all up to yous...We have a NEED to FEED !!!

Dirt; "the Lord God formed man of the dust of the ground..." (Genisis 2:7) & "of the ground made the Lord God to grow every tree that is pleasant sight and good for food..." (Genesis 2:9); which tells us that the soil is the key to sustainig us. It is true that the nutrition of, let's say, a tomato from South America is diffiernt from a tomato from North America is different from a tomato from Italy, especially from San Marzano, where there is volcanic ash...(It would probably be easier if we ate dirt; though, not so tasty)...

Just a few weeks ago, on a PBS station, I was watching a nature program and it showed chimpanzees, individually, walking up the a hollowed out tree, with an offering, a stone and placing their stone at the mouth of the tree, until they each had their turn. Then, they just sat there looking at the tree.

i sat there looking at the TV with the same look as (my cousins) the chimpanzees; yous know that look. like in the cartoon strips when the light bulb goes on over ones head or like when a dog is tilting it's head as if it's trying to pay attention to every word you're saying (rather than that snack, that's pictured over the dog's head)...

It was a Religious Ceremony (kinda silly, AHEY); like spinning bells, or kneeling and bowing, or proceeding to communion, or standing armpit deep in a cold river, or banging ones head against a wall... In the Gospels Jesus admonishes us to: "Love God and Love each other" (John 13:33-34); and we do anything, but...

The Good News (or Gospel for you students of Greek) is that things are not as dire as they use to be; just check one of your past life-times, to be sure... Maybe, because the Gospel of Grace is beginning to penetrate our hearts and minds; Maybe NOT...

Probably because of Democracy (a liberal thought), the affluence in the world is spreading to many who had not. At the start of the 1900's; 99% of the worlds population lived in abject poverty (defined as not knowing where one's next meal was coming from) and by the second millenium (the year 2000); 80% of the world's population lived in abject poverty. This means that the 20th century has been a true powerhouse on this Earth; even with a population increase of nearly three fold, nearly 20% more people were moved into a more comfortable life-style and responded in kind, with the explosion of Charities and Foundations to aid those least of us..."Whatever you do for the least of your brothers, that you do also for me"...(Jesus, circa 30 AD).

Looks like The Buddha was correct when he said the middle way is the best way...

So - How'd Yous Like Our Scavenger Hunt ??? Was it every thing I said it would be ??? So - What should we go after next ??? Noah's Ark ??? Na - that's been done over and over.

How's about the lost Years of Jesus ???

In the Gospels we see Jesus at his birth (from which he had to hi-tail-it outta town), at his Bar-Mitz-Va (at which he got lost) and when he began his ministry (he really should of hooked-up with a good - P.R. firm)...Well there is some talk that he may have wandered, after all, Jesus was a day laborer. He eventually figured out that it was a way lot better to accept money for saying nice stuff, than humping stones to built a wall, or help out at harvest time (mucho trabajo, poco dinero; translates - much work, little money).

Do yous think Jesus may have traveled ???

Maybe with a caravan to places unknown. Why Not ??? Maybe to Arabia...Jesus did speak Arimeic; the Koran is written in Arimeic... Maybe to India ??? Three hundred (some odd) years earlier, Alexander the Great, made a highway from Greece through Babylon to India...

In Luke 6:31, Jesus tells us -"do unto others, as you would have them do unto you"...This is the Law of Karma...Did he learn things in India that magnified his healing abilities ??? That would explain quite-a-bit...

What about - Genisis 3:23 -"So he drove out the man; and he placed at the east of the garden of Eden - Cherubims and a flaming sword which turned every way, to keep the way of the tree of life." (KJV)...Yeah, that's it - The Tree of Life... God, the Omnipotent, never destroys it (the Tree of Life); He chooses to preserve it. Instead of the dramatic - Turning Flaming Sword and the Cherubims (are they the cute baby-like ones without diapers ?) protecting the tree; God, could of just sizzled the tree. It would of made the point and Adam krap his loin-cloth...

Yeah -The TREE of LIFE !!! if I am still around in a few hundred years, then we will know - I figured it out !!! Yeaaa... This adventure begins - now...

BIBLIOGRAPHY

The word - bibliography, means a group of books compiled to contribute to a work; its root coming from the work - Bible, meaning a group of stories compiled to form a book and the word - Biblioteca, stems from this also meaning, library... The following is a listing of books that aided me in my thesis, along with those I would recommend for your reading to further deepen your knowledge upon this subject matter...

- Public Broadcast Service (PBS) stations
- authorized King James version of the Holy Bible
- the Good News Bible in today's english version
- the Bible, revised standard version
- the new American Bible
- the American Heritage Dictionary of the English Language
- Webster's Third New International dictionary (unabridged)
- Benjamin Franklin, an American Life by Walter Isaacson
- Gandhi by Louis Fischer
- The Life of Andrew Jackson by Robert V. Remini
- Cicero, the Life and Times by Anthony Everitt
- the Gospel of Philip by Jean-Yves LeLoup
- the Gospel of Mary of Magdala by Karen L, King
- the Secret Gospel according to Mark by Morton Smith
- The Illustrated Encyclopedia of Buddhist Wisdom by Gill Farrer-Halls
- Evolution of the Gods by Ajay Kansal
- 101 Myths of the Bible by Gary Greenberg

- Misquoting Jesus by Bart D. Ehrman
- The Truth about Muhammad by Robert Spencer
- The History of the Written Word by Kevin Cunningham
- the Double Helix by James Watson
- DNA the Secret of Life by James Watson
- The Ego and the Id by Dr. Sigmund Freud
- Mucusless Diet, a scientific method of eating your way healthy by Arnold Ehret
- Eat to Live by Joel Fuhrman, MD
- Eat Dirt by Dr. Josh Axe
- Fasting and Eating for Health by Joel Fuhrman, MD
- Naturopathic Nutrition by Abram Hiffer & Johnathen Prousky
- Nutrition for Intuition by Doreen Virtue & Robert Reeves
- Archangels & Ascended Masters by Doreen Virtue
- Unlock your Senventh Sense by Lucy Marcella
- Seven Universal Principles and the Seventh Sense by Dr. Nader Butto
- The Healing Power of Herbs by May Bethel
- The Most Effect Cures on Earth by Jonny Bowden, PHD
- Vitamin Book by Virginia DeMoss
- The Healing Nutrients Within by Eric Braverman, MD
- Deep Nutrition by Catherine Shanahan, MD & Luke Shanahan
- Putting it all Together, New Orthomolecuar Nutrition by Abram Hoffer, MD & Morton Walker
- Hippocrates: Making the Way for Medicne by Connie Jankowski
- The Hippocrates Diet and Health Program by Ann Wigmore

- The Macrobiotic Path to Health by Michio Kushi & Alex Jack
- Eat for Health by Joel Fuhrman, MD
- The 150 Healthiest Foods on Earth by Jonny Boeden, PHD
- The Eggplant Cancer Cure by Johnathan V. Wright, MD
- The ABC's of Hormones by Jack Challem
- Human Hormones by Books LLc.
- Hormones, Health, and Happiness by Steven F. Horze, MD
- Change your DNA Change your Health by Dr. Robert V. Gerard
- Amino Acids in Theraphy by Leon Chaitow, DO, ND
- Thorson's Guide to Amino Acids by Leon Chaitow, ND, DO
- The Amino Revolution by Robert Erdmann, Phd
- Enzymes, the Key to Health by Howard F. Loomis Jr., DC
- Enzymes, Enzyme Theraphy by Dr. Anthony J. Cichoke
- Enzyme Nutrition by Dr. Edward Howell
- Enzymes, the Fountain of Life by D.A.Lopez, MD; R.M.Williams, MD & M.Miehlke, MD
- The Nature of Animal Healing by Martin Goldstein, DVM
- Depression Free Naturally by Joan Mathews Larson, Phd
- Nature's Law, the secret of the Universe by R.N.Elliott
- The Immortality Edge by Michael Fossel, MD;Greta Blackburn & Dave Woynarowski, MD
- Pottenger's Prophecy by Cary Graham, NTP;Deborah Kesten, MPH;Larry Scherwitz, Phd

- Breads, Manna feom Heaven by Eileen Gaden
- Baking with Quinoa by Sarah Clarence
- The Everything Sprouted Grains Book by Brandi Evans
- Sproutman's Kitchen garden cookbook by Steve Meyerowitz
- Encyclopedia of Nuts, berrie and seeds by John Heinerman
- New Encyclopedia of fruits & vegetables by John Heinerman
- The Winter Harvest Handbook by Eliot Coleman
- The Vegetable Gardener's Container Bible by Edward C. Smith
- The Little Prince by Antoine de Saint-Exupery

www.ingramcontent.com/pod-product-compliance
Lightning Source LLC
Chambersburg PA
CBHW050924260726
48660CB00001B/381